OXFORD MEDICAL PUBLICATIONS

Anatomy of a Hospital

Anatomy of a Hospital

JULIAN ASHLEY

Oxford   Melbourne   Toronto
OXFORD UNIVERSITY PRESS
1987

Oxford University Press, Walton Street, Oxford OX2 6DP

Oxford New York Toronto
Delhi Bombay Calcutta Madras Karachi
Petaling Jaya Singapore Hong Kong Tokyo
Nairobi Dar es Salaam Cape Town
Melbourne Auckland

and associated companies in
Beirut Berlin Ibadan Nicosia

Oxford is a trade mark of Oxford University Press

Published in the United States
by Oxford University Press, New York

British Library Cataloguing in Publication Data
Ashley, Julian
Anatomy of a hospital.—(Oxford medical
publications).
1. Hospitals—Great Britain
I. Title
362.1'1'0941   RA986
ISBN 0-19-261578-5

Library of Congress Cataloging in Publication Data
Ashley, Julian.
Anatomy of a hospital.
(Oxford medical publications)
Includes index.
1. Hospitals, Teaching—Great Britain.   2. Medical
care—Great Britain.   I. Title.   II. Series. [DNLM:
1. Hospital Administration—popular works.   Hospitals—
popular works.   WX 150 A826a]
RA986.A88   1988   362.1'1'0942   87-15399
ISBN 0-19-261578-5

Set by Cambrian Typesetters, High Street, Frimley, Surrey.
Printed in Great Britain
at the University Printing House Oxford
by David Stanford
Printer to the University

PREFACE

This book is written by someone who has worked in hospitals for 30 years and who is still excited by them. At any moment of the day or night, year in and year out, hundreds of intense personal dramas are simultaneously unfolding in any large general hospital. Sadness and joy, pain and relief, earnest discussions about difficult cases, simple words of comfort, and miracles of sophistication are the endlessly recurring experiences of patients, staff, and relatives in wards and clinics, operating theatres and diagnostic departments, accident and emergency receiving rooms, corridors, and interviewing rooms all over the building.

The building is the Royal Infirmary, a hospital which does not exist and which at the same time is as accurate a portrait of a great provincial teaching hospital as it is possible to construct. Any institution of such complexity is bound to present paradoxes. The Royal Infirmary is shabby, impersonal, uncomfortable, expensive, and inefficient. At the same time, it is overworked, underfunded, and perpetually striving against overwhelming odds to meet the ever increasing demands made upon it by the persistently unhealthy citizens of the District. Wonderful work goes on within its walls, where the training and discipline of the staff and the advances in medical technology are locked in perpetual battle with the ageing of the population. Waiting lists for many routine operations are long, and the notice given to patients to come in is short. No wonder it enjoys a love–hate relationship with both its customers and its staff, and evokes passionate loyalty and bitter resentment from press and public alike. The Royal Infirmary does not exist, so it had to be invented. The names and the personalities referred to bear no relationship to any patient or any member of the medical or nursing professions. The Infirmary is a mixture of innumerable hospitals throughout the country, part District General, part Regional Centre, part teaching hospital. I have attempted to present as many of its facets as possible, and only regret that I have had to leave unsung so many of its heroes and heroines who are making vital contributions to patient care in departments I have been unable to visit, often because they are small and highly specialized. Those departments to which I have been able to make scant reference or none at all include the dental surgeons, the chaplains, social work, speech therapy, orthoptics, cytogenetics, tissue typing, immunology, electro-encephalography, and medical illustration. In addition, I plead guilty to the use of what may appear to be sexist language: it is simply easier to refer to the doctor as 'he' and the nurse as 'she' and it interrupts the flow to keep on using the correct but clumsy 'he or she'.

Finally, it has become dangerously fashionable in the politics of healthcare to scorn big institutions and to regard 'the Community' as a universal panacea. The distinction is a spurious one. The hospital exists to serve its community, and if it is not a part of that community it is nothing.

JULIAN ASHLEY

CONTENTS

ABBREVIATIONS

A&E	Accident and Emergency
AIDS	Acquired immune deficiency syndrome
ALAC	Artificial Limb and Appliance Centre
ANC	Ante-natal clinic
BID	Brought in dead
BMA	British Medical Association
BMJ	*British Medical Journal* (organ of the BMA)
BP	Blood pressure
BS	Batchelor of Surgery
CABG	Coronary artery bypass grafting
CAPD	Continuous ambulatory peritoneal dialysis
CCU	Coronary care unit
CHC	Community Health Council
CHD	Coronary heart disease
COHSE	Confederation of Health Service Employees
CPC	Clinico-pathological conference
CPR	Cardio-pulmonary resuscitation
CSSD	Central sterile supplies department
CT (CAT)	Computed tomography (Computerized axial tomography)
c.v.	Curriculum vitae
D&C	Dilatation and curettage (of womb)
DDC	Drug dependency clinic
DGH	District General Hospital
DHA	District Health Authority
DHSS	Department of Health and Social Security
DMB	District Management Board
DPC (or U)	Drinking problem clinic (or unit)
DSA	Digital subtraction angiography
DU	Duodenal ulcer
ECG	Electrocardiogram
ECT	Electroconvulsive therapy
EEG	Electroencephalogram
ENB	English National Board (of nursing)
ENT	Ears, nose, and throat
ERCP	Endoscopic retrograde cholangio-pancreatography
FBC	Full blood count
FFARCS	Fellow of the Faculty of Anaesthetists of the RCS
FIMLS	Fellow of the Institute of Medical Laboratory Scientists

FRCP	Fellow of the Royal College of Physicians
FRCS	Fellow of the Royal College of Surgeons
GMC	General Medical Council
GP	General practitioner (family physician)
GU	Gastric ulcer
HAA	Hospital Activity Analysis
HIPE	Hospital in-patient enquiry
HP, HS	House physician, house surgeon
i.m. (i)	Intramuscular (injection)
ITU, ICU	Intensive therapy (or treatment or care) unit
i.v (i)	Intravenous (injection, infusion)
£1K	£1000
LFT	Liver function tests
MB	Batchelor of Medicine
MD	Doctor of Medicine
MI	Myocardial infarction ('heart attack')
MLSO	Medical laboratory scientific officer
MPS	Member of the Pharmaceutical Society
MRC	Medical Research Council
MRCP	Member of the Royal College of Physicians
MRI	Magnetic resonance imaging (formerly termed nuclear magnetic resonance or NMR)
NHS	National Health Service
NUPE	National Union of Public Employees
O&G	Obstetrics and gynaecology
ODA	Operating department assistant
OT	Occupational therapy or therapist
PHLS	Public Health Laboratory Service
PM	Post-mortem
QALY	Quality adjusted life year
RCN	Royal College of Nursing
RCP	Royal College of Physicians
RCS	Royal College of Surgeons
RC (GP, O&G, Path, Psych, R)	Royal Colleges (General Practitioners, Obstetricians and Gynaecologists, Pathologists, Psychiatrists, Radiologists)
RGN	Registered General Nurse
RHA	Regional Health Authority
RI	Royal Infirmary
RMN	Registered Mental Nurse
RTA	Road traffic accident
RTD	Radiotherapy department
SCBU	Special care baby unit
SEN	State Enrolled Nurse

SHO	Senior house officer
SR	Senior registrar
SRN	State Registered Nurse
STD	Sexually transmitted diseases
T&O	Trauma and orthopaedics
TSSU	Theatre sterile supply unit
TURP	Trans-urethral resection of prostate
U&E	Urea and electrolytes
UGC	University Grants Committee
UKCC	UK Central Council for Nursing, Midwifery and Health Visiting
UTI	Urinary tract infection
VDU	Visual display unit
VTS	Vocational training scheme (usually for general practice)
WTE	Whole-time equivalent (e.g. nurse)

1

The hotel

The last half-hour of the train journey from London is pleasant enough to make the traveller look up from his book or paper from time to time just in case he is missing anything dramatic. However, the undulating expanses of immaculate arable land continue to flow past uninterrupted except by the occasional defiantly surviving hedge. Even in early summer the only variation in the endless green ocean is the startling intrusion of a vivid yellow slick of oil-seed rape. Then, due to no apparent change in the passing scene, the urgency fades almost imperceptibly from the train's headlong charge, there is a rustling of papers and a clicking of briefcases, and outside the crops give way to geometrical estates of red brick houses with here and there one or two small warehouses. The main industrial area is the other side of the city, decently shielded from the middle-class eyes of the south-east of the county. Passengers on the left-hand side who are not . too busy putting on their coats and reaching for their cases will be struck by the white cliffs of the new Royal Infirmary (RI), which tower abruptly above the surrounding suburbs. When construction started during the early-1960s, it was on the edge of the city, but it has since been engulfed by its local populace who look to it for work and for care, rather like a medieval castle surrounded by tenants who defend it and in turn seek its protection. The first time I made this journey was in 1971, and at that time the forbidding but familiar jigsaw of Victorian masonry that was the old Royal Infirmary still provided most of the day-to-day hospital services of the city. It was much more convenient in many ways, because the town was then of manageable proportions and the railway station, the cathedral, the shopping centre and the hospital were all within a few minutes walk of each other. Even the factories and the university campus, dating from the early-1930s, were only a bicycle ride or a couple of bus stops away. The new hospital has developed and expanded prodigiously over the past 16 years. The pace of that expansion was accelerated by the development of the new medical school in the early-1970s, and the consultant staff which was about 45 strong when I joined it has swollen to some 170 members. With the closure of the old RI in 1983, almost all the hospital services became concentrated on the one site. It is that site which forms the theme of this book, for the RI is in many ways typical of a number of large teaching hospitals and has many roles and an astonishing range of activities.

The RI is certainly the largest and most valuable building in the city, and easily dwarfs Her Majesty's Prison, which must be the runner-up. It stands on a prime site of some 70 acres contained within a perimeter road with two main points of access from the surrounding streets. The buildings form a complex rather like the Himalayas with the eight snowy concrete storeys of the main ward block as Everest towering above the lower ranges formed by the medical school, the school of nursing, the residences, and the doctors' mess, with a number of ground level extensions sprawled around as the foothills. The structure contains 10 million bricks (enough to build an estate of 900 houses) together with sufficient concrete for 70 miles (112 km) of road. There are 2½ miles (4 km) of corridor, 12 000 rooms and a covered floor area totalling 55 acres, and the area of glass is almost 15 acres. The whole complex must be worth £25 million. It takes skilled workers to operate the plant and maintain the fabric of such a massive enterprise, and about 80 plumbers, electricians, and engineers are employed full time to keep the place running. There are also three or four gardeners, although the lawns and flower-beds are retreating before the inexorable advance of car parks and laboratories. In fact, one of the gardeners has undergone a conversion course to become a sort of amateur pest control officer and spends most of his time disposing of the kittens spawned by the feral cats which roam the grounds and the basement, and which help him to keep the mice, rats, pigeons, and sparrows within reasonable limits. The old RI used to have a pigeon problem and the mites would breed in their nests and fall through the rafters onto the patients, occasionally causing spectacular crops of bites.

Today a hospital costs £15 000–£20 000 (£15K–£20K) a bed to build, but this includes extensive additional accommodation for laboratories, offices, and out-patient suites. The fashion in most Continental countries has long favoured a large number of small rooms, either individual or shared by two, three, or four patients. The 34 wards of the RI are similar to those in most modern British hospitals, and are divided into three open bays containing six beds each to facilitate observation by the nursing staff, together with four single cubicles where potentially infectious patients can be nursed. There is also a two-bed room and a four-bedder, making 28 beds on a typical ward, and a modest day-room.

So much for the bricks and mortar: what about the upkeep? To start with, a hospital consumes a vast amount of power, and the RI's electricity bill mounts up at a rate of over £2 a minute during the winter months. The current is conveyed throughout the premises by 930 miles (1500 km) of cable. The five gas-fired boilers are each the size of a garage and heating the establishment costs up to about £3 a minute but 32 000 gallons (145 000 litres) of oil are kept in tanks on site as standby fuel. The works department is in charge of over 10 000 rooms separated from each other and from the corridors and the outside world by more than 12 500 doors. There are 58 lifts, there are water storage tanks with more than a quarter of a million gallons (1 125 000 litres) capacity, the Rolls Royce motors can generate 1700 kilowatts in 30 seconds, and the refrigeration plant can produce over 200 tons of ice an hour. The incinerator can accept 1111 lbs (500 kg) of waste at a time and operates at up to 1200 °C, and the quantity of steel which the department embraces would construct a couple of frigates for the Navy. The daily water consumption is 120 000 gallons (545 500 litres) conducted through 150 miles (240 km) of pipe.

These great edifices are highly dependent on the mains services. A consultant at a teaching hospital in the south-east told me of the exploits of Sedgwick the cat. At about 6 o'clock on a dreary February evening in the early-1980s, a sudden power failure extinguished all the lights of the southern half of the city and the surrounding villages. Normally, the hospital's own generators should immediately and automatically take over, but on this occasion the mechanism was put to the test and failed. Luckily, only one patient was being artificially ventilated (respirated) at the time, and there was little problem about continuing this manually until the power was restored a few hours later. One of the lifts became stuck between floors, and all the vacuum cleaners which were being used to clean the carpets in the entrance hall of the out-patients department after the day's wear and tear, came to a sudden halt. The cleaning staff promptly walked out, with the result that when the electricity came on again shortly after nine, the hallway was filled with the pandemonium of seven vacuum cleaners charging about driverless, getting their flexes in a twist and colliding with each other and with pieces of furniture. Somebody said it was probably a prowling fox which had inadvertently stepped on some poorly insulated cables at the power station, but no fox was to be seen. A day or two later, Sedgwick, an elderly ginger cat who had been missing for three days, returned home looking and smelling, according to his doting owners, like a burnt tyre. He was clearly feeling very sorry for himself, the vet said that his injuries looked like an electric burn, and letters poured in wishing him a speedy recovery. These wishes were fulfilled and Sedgwick was not only none the worse for his experience, but his

habitual mild melancholia lifted completely in dramatic response to his short
course of electroconvulsive therapy.

Of its many roles, the RI is first and foremost a District General
Hospital (DGH) and serves the people of its own Health District. Its
catchment population is about 370 000, about half of whom live
within the city and the remainder in the surrounding villages and
market towns of the county. It is not entirely self-sufficient since one
or two smallish towns on the edge of our empire traditionally look
towards neighbouring health districts. Also, the old psychiatric
hospital, situated in what used to be an attractive village but has since
been engulfed into a charmless suburban sprawl, still copes with the
great majority of mental illness requiring admission to hospital, since
the construction of a psychiatric unit on the RI site remains a long
overdue development. In addition, there is an old workhouse, also on
the other side of town, still in service as a geriatric hospital for aged
persons unfortunate enough to remain dependent on nursing care.
The RI is also a Regional Centre and provides much of the
sophisticated technology beyond the means of an ordinary DGH for
the inhabitants of the neighbouring three counties which are also
included in our Region. It is inextricably linked with the medical
school and is thus a vital part of the university. It is a training school
for nurses and physiotherapists and provides postgraduate training in
a wide range of disciplines.

Perhaps before it can do any of these things it has to be an 'hotel'.
Indeed, the original function of a hospital was basically that of an
hotel but with a religious or charitable rather than commercial
purpose. The 750 little hospitals of medieval England existed to offer
hospitality and shelter to wayfarers, pilgrims, and the needy, although
some specifically existed to house and isolate the lepers who were
abundant in England until the sixteenth century. Today, the clients of
the hotel are the patients—950 of them. The size is worth a comment.
In 1959 there were 28 hospitals in England with over 2000 beds, but
by 1980 the 'small is beautiful' ideology had influenced the mandarins
of Whitehall almost as profoundly as had the economic performance
of the nation, and none were left. Indeed, there were only 10 non-
psychiatric hospitals with over 1000 beds, although other advanced
countries seem to find large hospitals perfectly manageable. So ours,
as British hospitals go (and there are over 600 within the National
Health Service, NHS), and certainly as hotels go, is a big one. Unlike
many hotels, there are no off-seasons and throughout the year the RI
operates to an occupancy rate of rather over 80 per cent. A moment's

thought will be sufficient to appreciate the impossibility of running an acute hospital with anything like 100 per cent of the beds full, for patients are being discharged all the time and the acutely sick can only be admitted into beds which have been vacated. Similarly, a figure much below the occupancy quoted would indicate that the hospital was under-used and that there were plenty of empty beds waiting for customers, a situation seldom if ever encountered in the NHS. Hotel services are required not only by the patients but also by the staff. Almost 800 of the 1600 nurses and 100 of the 400 doctors occupy the somewhat bleak residences and therefore use the catering, cleaning, and laundry facilities. In addition, a large number of all grades of staff takes lunch in the main canteen. There is, therefore, an army of workers employed to man the essential departments and most of them are employed on a more-or-less nine to five, Monday to Friday basis with a skeleton staff providing meals at weekends and for the night nurses. On weekdays, about 3500 workers flock through the main entrance of the hospital grounds, and since the city's bus services have been allowed to run down over the past couple of decades, most of them come by car. This is one of the management's more intractable problems. Numerous private cars arrive during the course of the day bringing 1000 out-patients up to the clinics, and a further motorcade brings visitors during the afternoon and evening. Thus, an educated guess would be that there are altogether about 10 000 people on the campus during any weekday afternoon—more of a small town rather than an hotel. No hospital has yet been built in the United Kingdom with adequate car parking facilities and the RI with its 1250 parking spaces, compared with an estimated requirement of 2000, is no exception. So instead, one of the porters tours the grounds slapping No Parking notices on vehicles parked on double yellow lines or in the restricted parking zones. A brief flirtation with wheel clamps was hurriedly dropped when violence erupted and the porters threatened to withdraw their services. Until the 1960s, it was taken for granted that VIPs such as consultants, the house governor, the matron, would automatically have their own named parking slots, but egalitarianism has swept the land, the latter two offices are long defunct, the consultants have multiplied, and now there are only a few parking areas restricted to various grades of staff and none which are personal.

The housekeeping staff are the least skilled and the poorest paid workers on the site, and the basic weekly rate of pay is about £87. There are 70 porters, 90 caterers, 350 domestics, and 60 laundry workers. They mainly belong to the National Union of Public Employees (NUPE) and the Confederation of Health Service Employees (COHSE), and from time to time become engaged in industrial disputes with the management. One of the thorny issues which continues to provoke much unrest is the privatization of cleaning, catering, and laundry services which has been enthusiastically promoted by Margaret Thatcher's government on the grounds that commercial enterprises can undertake these functions more economically than an 'in-house' workforce, thereby relieving the health service management of direct negotiations with the unions. Economies have undoubtedly been effected, although often at the expense of jobs and sometimes at the expense of standards.

The 'hotel' industry of the NHS is big business, albeit run on a shoestring. Prices quoted throughout this book are mid-1980s levels: and the catering cost for a patient for a day is £3–4 of which food currently accounts for £1.95. It may be mentioned that we are in the happy position of being able to buy our beef at little more than a quarter (50p a pound, 0.45 kg) of the usual price through 'intervention' supplies—the EEC 'mountain'. The vegetables are delivered already prepared by a contract wholesaler. The amount of tea purchased by the District Health Authority each year is 800 kg. The kitchen of the RI, which is the largest in the city, produces some 4500 meals per day. Those for the patients are cooked centrally, put on trays by a couple of assembly lines in accordance with the menu cards filled in by the patients the previous day, and wheeled by the porters in large insulated trolleys to the wards where they are dispensed by the nurses. Hospital food is criticized by the patients because they do not like it and because they are unable to tell which out of the choices of three or four main courses and a similar number of puddings available they are likely to fancy the following day—which does not matter much because they seldom get what they ordered anyway. It is criticized by staff because there has been, until very recently, insufficient input by the dieticians who should be very much involved in planning what is, after all, a most important part of the patients' overall health care. It is not in accordance with current dietary thinking, for example, that 280 lb (126 kg) of chips are cooked for lunch and 140 lb (63 kg) for supper. In addition, 350–400 rolls are consumed each day, few of which are made of wholemeal bread. Enormous quantities of this food, probably several tons a week, are wasted, and whether or not the diet is appropriately health-conscious for patients, it certainly seems to nourish the local pigs pretty well.

Being a customer of the hotel is not much fun, even if you are not feeling rotten and no one is doing unpleasant things to you. My advice is to put your watch forward by two hours as you enter the emporium of healing. It is usual to be woken up at 6.30 a.m., and to receive your breakfast in or by your bed shortly afterwards. Locally, we gave up eggs and bacon in favour of a Continental breakfast a couple of years ago. The early morning medicine round adds to the bustle of activity, and is followed by bathing for those who need it. Then boredom, punctuated (unpleasantly) by treatment or (briefly) by doctors' rounds until lunch at 11.45 a.m. More medicines, a rest hour, visitors, and tea—and then the last meal at about 6 p.m. High tea? Low dinner? Fortunately for those feeling well enough to become rather peckish later in the evening, the wards have little kitchens where the staff will prepare a sandwich and a warm drink at about 8 p.m. After that, if you have taken my advice concerning the difference between GMT and RI time, it seems a reasonable hour at which to turn in.

The laundry is the busiest in the city. Sheets are changed in theory every week, but in practice much more often, when a new patient takes over the bed, or when the occupant vomits or fouls the bed or gushes blood all over it or spills his lunch into it. About 120 000–150 000 items are laundered each week. Many of the patients have not arrived suitably equipped because of failure to anticipate, for example, that their drive down the motorway would terminate in carnage, so towel, toothpaste, and nightclothes have to be provided as well. While on the subject of sanitation, it might be mentioned that the whole complex is thought to contain 3500 lavatories and that the supplies officer issues 121 000 toilet rolls (about 400 km of paper) a year. The myriad of items needed to keep the place running are held in the supplies department which is a vast subterranean Aladdin's cave. In it you can find anything and everything: syringes, stationery, bandages, apples, shrouds, cans of Guinness, as well as all those toilet rolls. There are 2760 regular stock lines and at least another 2000 items not held in stock but frequently purchased. The value at any one time is at least £500K, and £180K worth is issued every month. Each month £9K is spent on stationery alone. One depressing but overwhelming impression from a stroll round the shelves is how few of the items originate or are manufactured in the United Kingdom—not even the apples. There are plans to centralize medical and surgical supplies by providing a regional depot in an aircraft hangar of a building on the new industrial estate of a market town 40 miles away.

This is generally viewed as a bad thing and a threat to the RI's autonomy.

There is no sharp distinction between the personnel who are involved in direct patient care and those who keep the establishment ticking over, and the telephonists are important members of both categories. There are 12 of them, at least two on duty at any one time, and most of them work shifts to cover calls around the clock. There are seven positions at the switchboard and the staff is augmented from 8.30 a.m. to 5.30 p.m. to fill as many positions as possible during office hours. Nevertheless, there are constant complaints at the delays experienced by frustrated General Practitioners (GPs) and relatives, since the system is simply not adequate to handle the 5000–10 000 incoming and outgoing calls made daily. There are 1100 extensions and by dailling 333 internally you can access the air-call or paging system and talk into someone's bleep and give him or her a short message. Even this arrangement is suffering from inflation, with about 200 members of staff of all categories regarding them as a sort of badge of indispensability and glamour—or as unpardonable intruders into the tranquillity of the lavatory.

Finally, no account of this vast organization would be complete without some mention of two professionals whose roles are crucial yet lonely ones, since their teams each consist of the proverbial one man and a dog. The first is the fire-officer, and he must assess and report on the possible fire hazards of any proposed development from a new building to a trial of duvets instead of conventional bedclothes. He also investigates all episodes of fire and in addition gives the fire lectures that each and every member of staff is supposed to attend annually. These lectures are intended to heighten awareness and are exceedingly effective in dispelling the 'it couldn't happen here' attitude which might otherwise prevail. Mercifully, there has been no catastrophic hospital fire in this country for many years, but not very long ago a major Brazilian psychiatric hospital was almost gutted with considerable loss of life and that tragedy grimly brought home the potential horror of fire in a high-rise building full of the sick and incapacitated as well as the able-bodied whose task it is to rescue them. There are 40–45 fires a year in the city's hospitals, the majority occurring in the psychiatric hospital. There are three times that number of false alarms, partly through the persistence of a psychiatric patient whose chief delight it is to see the fire brigade in action, but often due to malfunction of the smoke detectors. At the RI there are 190 fire zones, where the alarm will sound in response to a smoke detector or to the act of breaking the glass with the hammer provided. The alarm also sounds in the telephone exchange, but they should also be directly contacted on a special number and will then notify the fire service as well as despatching the fire officer and two or three other key people to the scene of the conflagration.

The hospital security officer has an office which is appropriately unidentifiable behind a blanket-grey door devoid of any indication of what lies within. Inside, a grizzled, burly ex-policeman in his mid-fifties towers over a desk hemmed in by cupboards full of hooks supporting well over 1000 keys. Like the fire officer, he is very much a one-man band, and therefore something of a voice crying in the wilderness. He admits that here, in the city, we are very lucky compared with London and many another metropolis—but that we are probably living in a fools' paradise:

We have perhaps a couple of thefts reported a week, most of them petty pilfering but during the past two or three years we have lost three microwave cookers, four TV sets, and two VDUs. This kind of item is usually stolen to order and when you are dealing with professionals, bolts and chains are virtually useless. So far, we haven't had to cope with a great deal of violence, but over the Christmas holiday we usually hire an officer from the local constabulary for the A and E department between 10 p.m. and 2 a.m. to protect the nurses and the casualty officers from violent drunks. You see, it takes a police car seven to nine minutes to get here if we have to call one.

We do get some very odd characters skulking around the hospital especially in the basement and on the ground floor. The undercroft is particularly poorly lit and full of rather sinister deserted areas and the nurses don't much care for some of the long corridors linking the hospital to the residences. It's not only the local villains but school kids during the holidays and unemployed youths, and also, of course, the dossers. We get quite a few of those, they come in especially during the winter months and kip down in deserted corners or in the boiler house if they can get in. You can't blame them, really, there isn't anywhere much else for them to go.

We haven't had any drugs stolen because our precautions are pretty well watertight, but I always give the student nurses a bit of a pep talk. They quite often get approached by people in the town at discos and places like that who try to prevail on them to obtain supplies for them. I want them to report that sort of incident at once. And the other thing I tell them is that it doesn't matter a toss if they drop an ampoule of morphine or heroin by mistake—it only costs a few pence to the hospital and it's only when it gets out onto the street that its price rockets. So as long as they report it to Sister, and don't just tidy it up, because if they do that there'll be an ampoule not accounted for and the whole investigative machinery will be set in motion.

This, then, is the environment into which the patients are received. The bricks and mortar, heating, lighting, and plumbing, are usually taken for granted. However, these activities that go on behind the scenes are in their way as essential for the treatment of the patients as are those of the doctors, nurses, and therapists with whom they come into contact.

2

The doctors

It would be ridiculous to claim that nothing changes on the day you pass your finals: an awful lot of things do. You apply for a job, you get paid, you have duties and responsibilities, you start being a qualified doctor. You do not, however, stop being a student. Whatever branch of medicine is ultimately chosen it will probably be another five–eight years of training and for those who specialize, at least one further stiff examination before you become established in your final career post. Even then, there is the continual need to keep reading, keep attending meetings, keep discussing with colleagues, so that everyone entering medical school is a lifelong student of medicine. There are broadly speaking, then, two groups of doctors on the staff of any hospital, the consultants and the training grades.

However, it should first of all be mentioned that the most important providers of medical care in and around the city are the 150 GPs now mainly grouped in some 40 or 45 three–six person partnerships who refer their patients to the various hospital departments. They do not, very often, come and see their patients in hospital because in-patients tend to be so inaccessible, always being down in the X-ray department or having physiotherapy, but they do come to various meetings in the hospital and some of them work one or two sessions a week assisting the various consultants.

The hospital medical staff proper is divided into about 170 consultants and 230 juniors and on the whole the former usually stay in the same appointment until they retire but the latter are birds of passage, holding successively higher appointments for successively longer durations in hospitals around the country until they too eventually achieve consultant rank. The other main difference, apart from age and salary, is that even if for some reason a particular patient never actually sees him, everyone admitted to hospital is under the overall care of a consultant who carries the final responsibility for treatment carried out by his juniors.

In order to practise medicine it is necessary to be on the medical register, and the newly-qualified doctor becomes provisionally registered, pending the satisfactory completion of his pre-registration year, when he can become fully registered. This year is spent in two periods of six months, one as a house physician and one as a house surgeon. It is increasingly common for each period to be further subdivided so that perhaps three months is spent in one of the medical specialties and three months in another. This period is traditionally something of a baptism of fire, though much less so than it was in the bad old days. During my own six months as house physician to a singularly evil-tempered consultant I was allowed only one Saturday morning off to be best man at a wedding. The thanks I received for this unremitting service were scant. 'These patients', observed the great man to the world at large in the middle of a ward round, 'must think I'm a bloody idiot to have a houseman like you'. In the face of such devastatingly well thought out abuse there are two courses open: join the French Foreign Legion or develop a thick skin. In return, I probably saved the old man's life on one occasion when he was stampeding about the minute office we all shared in one of his ungovernable tantrums and barged against a wardrobe on top of which a heavy filing cabinet was precariously balanced. At my instinctive cry, he leapt aside with surprising agility as the cabinet crashed to the ground. The senior registrar, who had been hoping for promotion for many years, never forgave me, but then it was the boss and not he on whom I relied for a reference. One of my contemporaries had the traumatic experience of being present when his equally cantankerous chief suffered a cardiac arrest. 'You should have waited five minutes and then carried out resuscitation' a colleague remarked. 'I did, I did', he replied, 'but it's impossible to tell if he's sustained irreversible brain damage or not'.

We live in more enlightened, if less colourful times, and today's houseman is probably on duty every second, third, or even fourth night. He is also, it might be added, significantly more likely to be a houseperson, since over 40 per cent of doctors qualifying are female. As one ascends the hospital hierarchy, this proportion thins out, until only 12 per cent of consultants are women (Table 2.1). There is a number of reasons for this, of which male chauvinism is the least important. There were fewer female medical students when today's consultants trained than there are now (the cohort effect). A career in hospital medicine requires total commitment and is difficult to reconcile with absences for child-birth and child rearing. Further-more, the aspiring specialist has to 'follow his star' which means moving around seeking the best job you can get—and in any partnership only one can lead the way while the other has to be towed around in the wake.

TABLE 2.1. Percentage of female doctors over a 10–year period (UK)

Female doctors	1974	1984
General practice	12	20
Hospital medicine	15	23
House officers	26	38
Senior house officers	20	30
Registrars	17	22
Senior registrars	18	25
Consultants	8	12
Consultant psychiatrists	–	25
Consultant general surgeons	–	2

(Student entry: 50 as from 1985)

Source: Bewley, Beulah, R. (1986). Women Doctors and the Medical Manpower Crisis. *British Journal of Hospital Medicine*, **36**, 237.

To return to the houseman's daily round, he is very much a prisoner in his ward and is fully occupied clerking in new admissions, arranging their investigations and treatment, dealing with every new crisis as it arises, and passing on information about the patients to his seniors. There are also endless forms to fill in—investigation requests, prescription charts, discharge notes to the GP, consultation requests to other consultants, and physiotherapy requests. The clerking process involves reading the GP's referral letter, which may be detailed or extremely scanty depending on the degree of emergency and the time of day, extracting the previous medical problems from the old case notes, if any, and sitting down with the patient and recording the features of the present complaint, unless the patient is *in extremis* and unable to describe them. This is followed by a full examination and all this information is recorded in the notes and preliminary diagnostic tests and treatment are initiated. The relatives have to be informed of the probable diagnosis and plan of action and any necessary instructions must be passed on to the nurses. For a given admission, all this may take up to an hour, and on a medical ward there may be three or four admissions on an average day. There are also practical things to do to patients. At the end of his year, the houseman will be adept at passing a catheter, putting up a drip, obtaining a sample of cerebrospinal fluid, tapping fluid from a chest or abdomen, recording an electrocardiogram, and inserting a central venous line. Once a week or so and occasional weekends the team is 'on-take' which means that those emergencies not referred to a specific consultant but either sent in via accident and emergency (A&E) or from the GP to the on-take team will come under its care, and then there may well be 15–20 or more admissions during the 24 hours. A number of them will be acutely and seriously sick, or even unconscious and need immediate action rather than the methodical approach just described, and usually a more senior member of the firm will see each patient briefly after the houseman (or instead of the houseman if they all come at once), and he will sort out those who present difficult problems. The consultant on take does not practise a great deal of 'sharp end' medicine at the RI although most of them do an evening round and will expect to be called in if a colleague should be admitted, not because of any greater competence than the senior registrar but out of personal concern. The consultant physician on take at my own teaching hospital was known as the physician of the day or POD: the surgeon of the day was very reluctant to submit to abbreviation, although the gynaecologist of the day had no such objections at all. The kind of emergencies that form the bread-and-butter work of a general medical team are pneumonia, stroke, heart attack, heart failure, asthma, drug overdose, and bleeding into the gut. On a general surgical firm the list would mainly consist of abdominal emergencies: appendicitis, strangulated hernia, perforated ulcer, and obstructed intestine. The firms at the RI each have a ward and consist of two teams, each with a house officer and a consultant, but sharing a single senior house officer, a registrar, and a senior registrar. The two consultants are independent of each other and some pairs get along well and others never meet but suspiciously count up the beds their opposite number is currently occupying.

At the RI, the two house physicians on each ward take it in turn to be on duty for nights and weekends which makes it quite hard going when one is on-take. The night is liable to be an interrupted one at the best of times, because the night nurses will ring the duty doctor if one of the patients gives cause for alarm or an intravenous line comes out of the vein and 'tissues' or they are not clear about a prescription—or a patient dies. During a busy night on take, the house physician probably will not go to bed at all.

In some of the newer non-teaching District General Hospitals, the structure is different and senior registrars in particular are becoming comparatively rare outside the teaching hospitals. There, the consultants do a great deal of the on-call work and the surgeons frequently have to come in during the night to carry out complex and major .

operations on often very sick and poor-risk patients. In 1981, a Royal Commission on medical manpower under the chairmanship of labour MP Renée Short recommended that consultants should do much more day-to-day patient care in the NHS and suggested the creation of many more firms with just houseman and consultant. These recommendations have yet to be widely implemented for a number of reasons. In the teaching centres such as the RI, the consultants may not do a great deal of night work or weekend work in the hospital, thanks to their numerous and highly competent juniors, but in theory at least they make up for it by spending a great deal of spare time writing, researching, correcting examination scripts, and preparing lectures. The structure of the firm is also different in the more highly specialized departments (eyes, plastic surgery, orthopaedics, obstetrics) where there are no pre-registration doctors: the latter are confined to the mainstream activities of general medicine and general surgery. Even the so-called general physicians, however, tend to have their own specialized interests—gastro-enterology, endocrinology, kidney disease, etc.

It should perhaps be explained that the medical profession in the United Kingdom has three anomalies of nomenclature. One is the fairly well-known one that a surgeon, after studying for five years or more to become a doctor, drops the title and reverts to 'Mister' a few years later on attaining his surgical qualifications. The second is that the title of 'Doctor' is a spurious one in that the qualifying degree is that of Bachelor of Medicine, not Doctor of Medicine (as in most countries). Finally, the term 'physician' is in general use to describe a General Practitioner or any practising doctor other than a surgeon, while the profession itself uses it to denote a hospital specialist in internal diseases, or what in the United States would be called an internist. There is, it may be added, a time-honoured series of definitions of the various specialists. A psychiatrist, it is said, knows nothing and does nothing. The surgeon knows nothing but does everything. The physician knows everything but does nothing while the pathologist knows everything but is a bit too late.

The two pre-registration house jobs are generally arranged by computer. The medical school has an arrangement with a number of hospitals in the region as well as the RI whereby the jobs go to the boys. The boys—and girls—during the months before qualifying apply for the jobs that attract them, either because they have been taught by, and impressed by, the consultant, or because the job is prestigious, or seems appropriate to what they eventually plan to do, or because others have found the experience enjoyable or valuable (or both). The consultants concerned similarly indicate whether they would find the application acceptable, or even desirable, and the computer matches applicant with consultant to their mutual satisfaction. All the applicant has to do is to pass his finals. All the students from the RI find themselves jobs without too much trouble, and it is not until a year later that the spectre of medical unemployment emerges from the shadows. At this stage it is highly desirable to have a general idea of what sort of career is appealing. It used to be much easier to change direction later, but nowadays interviewers become somewhat annoyed when they learn that an applicant for a GP training appointment has only chosen to apply as a second best having been disappointed in his earlier intention to become a neurosurgeon. Almost 40 per cent of medical students express a preference for general practice, and indeed some 60–70 per cent of doctors eventually become GPs. After registration, they need to spend a further three years in training, one as a trainee in a practice and the other two as senior house officers (SHOs) in various relevant hospital departments—A&E, general medicine, geriatrics, obstetrics, psychiatry, etc. Those who wish to become surgeons will seek SHO posts on various surgical firms as well as A&E. They will need to learn the skills of surgery by apprenticeship. They will also need to take further examinations—the first and second parts of the Fellowship of the Royal College of Surgeons, the first part being back to the basic sciences, the second including examining patients in front of the examiners and discussing them, and oral examinations. The pass rate for each part is about 25–30 per cent but the examination can be resat every four months up to a maximum number of attempts at a cost of £100 for the first part and £200 for the second.

A Senior house officer is fractionally more senior than a houseman and is given a greater degree of responsibility, probably including sessions in the out-patient department. The appointment lasts six months, and after perhaps a couple of six month stints, provided that he is progressing satisfactorily, he can scan the advertisements in the *British Medical Journal* to see if there are any attractive registrar jobs to apply for. These last for a year, usually renewed for a further year. Senior house officer and registrar posts are increasingly being absorbed into locally-organized rotating training schemes for general medicine, general surgery, and general practice. One of the responsibilities which usually falls to the SHO or registrar is the acceptance of patients from the GP. When a GP of considerable seniority demands an urgent admission, it is impossible for an SHO just over a year qualified to refuse, particularly since the GP and the SHO's chief may well be golf partners of long standing. In any case, the GP has seen the patient and knows how ill he is so it is difficult to disagree or cross-examine him. However, the SHO, or the registrar, knows how tight the bed situation is, so perhaps he says 'send him along to the admissions unit and we'll take a look at him'. This provides an escape clause whereby if they decide that the pain is just an attack of indigestion and not a coronary, they can, if sufficiently brave, send the patient straight home again with some antacid. Otherwise, it is a question of finding a bed. In the case of a suspected coronary, this will be in the coronary care unit (CCU), but for other conditions it will be an ordinary ward—and if the admitting team do not have a bed on their ward, they have to borrow one from another medical firm, or even a surgical firm, which does little to foster good relationships and professional brotherhood: 'Alright, if you *must* lodge your patient with us, you must—but only until tomorrow, mind, we've got someone coming into that bed. And anyway, the last thing we want is your coughing, spitting chest problems on our nice clean surgical ward'.

The aspiring physician must take his higher qualification at the SHO or registrar level, and for him it is the membership examination of the Royal College of Physicians (RCP), again in two parts: basic science and clinical. The pass rate is perhaps fractionally lower than that of the Royal College of Surgeons (RCS) and, having sooner or later triumphed, a warm glow of pride and joy is entirely justified. It does not last long, however, because it is quickly followed by the realization that, so far from being a certificate of specialist competence, it is merely the entrance ticket to further training and that henceforth you are competing at a different level, that is, with others who are all also members of the RCP. Fellowship of the RCP, it should be added, comes years later—by a secret process of election following several years as a consultant. The path ahead is still full of obstacles: after being a registrar, it is necessary to compete for a highly sought after senior registrar post and to remain in that for about three years acquiring technical skills in some specialized field of medicine before starting to apply for consultant jobs. During the years following membership, it is also necessary to publish papers in the various medical journals. The value of a person's publications is judged by the prestige of the journals concerned—the *British Medical Journal* (*BMJ*), the *Lancet*, and one or two American journals rating fairly near the top with a whole host of others being less highly regarded. It is also judged by the content. Does it represent a solid piece of research or is it merely a report of an unusual case? Finally, was Dr X the sole author, the first-named of the three, or the last-named of 17 co-authors? Considering the fact that 800 000 original papers are published annually in the world's 20 000 medical journals (and the number continues to grow), it might be supposed that publication is an easy matter, but this is far from the truth and most editors accept only a small proportion of papers submitted and most authors receive several rejection slips before their cherished brain-child is accepted. In addition to his publications, it is becoming increasingly important for the future physician or surgeon to take a research degree. British universities, for instance, award the degree of doctor of medicine on the basis of a thesis which will probably be the result of two years of research, and this may involve a break in normal training to spend a year or two as a research registrar.

The Royal Colleges of Physicians and Surgeons in London have their counter-parts in Scotland and Ireland and also in Canada and the Antipodes. They are by no means the only medical Royal Colleges: the obstetricians and gynaecologists have their own, and so, more recently, have the pathologists, the psychiatrists, the radiologists, and the general practitioners—all offering highly-prized diplomas won through highly-priced ordeals. They all, it may be added, take themselves inordinately seriously.

The duties of a senior registrar are really six-fold. As well as direct patient care, he will be called upon to teach medical students and junior doctors and he will be expected to continue with some research and to involve himself in administration. He will 'act up' for the consultants for whom he works during absences, and his final duty is to himself—to prepare himself in every way to become a consultant.

My current Senior registrar, Marilyn (I call her Marilyn, she calls me Dr Ashley except on social occasions) has so far applied unsuccessfully for two consultant jobs. This is par for the course and she is not in the least discouraged. Each week she studies the advertisements and asks me what I know about the posts advertised, the facilities, the other consultants in the same specialty in the hospital concerned. Will I kindly supply a reference? Can she have a day off to go and look at the place and meet the people there? It may be that the physician is an old friend of mine. I take the opportunity to give him a ring and tell him what an outstanding person Marilyn has turned out to be. He tells me guardedly that they have a fine field of applicants—all with excellent c.vs., having done excellent jobs, all with masses of publications, most with MDs. It is going to be a bit difficult to draw up a short-list. Eventually five or six are called for interview. The selection panel has a lay chairman: it has two consultants from the same department in the hospital concerned: there is a university nominee: there is a Royal College of Physicians representative: and there are two or three other consultants and another lay member representing the Health Authority. Why does Marilyn wish to come and work for the rest of her life at St. Elsewhere's? What has she to offer that would make her the best choice for the job? Having seen the place, are there any changes she would wish to introduce into the department? What does she think about the current upheaval in the Health Service? The questions go on for 30–40 minutes. Finally, she has very patiently answered all the committee's questions, has she any to put to the committee? No, thank you, Dr Y supplied all the necessary details when she came to look at the place. Good, in that case perhaps she would be kind enough to wait with the other candidates while the committee spends the next hour and a half on the impossible task of selecting a *primum inter pares*. She withdraws. Tea and biscuits are circulated. References are read—all the interviewed candidates have been among the best SRs that their referees have ever had the pleasure of working with. All would make excellent choices for the job. Finally, the two consultants who will have to work with the appointed person have the last word and speak in favour of Marilyn. It is settled, to the committee's relief, to my relief, and most of all to Marilyn's relief. Has it been fair? Probably about as fair as possible, given the competition.

Any sexual discrimination must remain unspoken. Any racial discrimination must remain unspoken. The latter accusation is not uncommon. I have sat on numerous interviewing committees for all grades of post and in different capacities, and have never encountered racial discrimination. Cultural discrimination, perhaps: there is a widespread feeling that Asian medical schools are inferior to our own and also that patients have a right to a doctor who can communicate properly with them. We now have many ethnic Asians who go through our universities and medical schools and speak English as their mother tongue, and I have never seen the slightest evidence of prejudice against them on racial grounds.

The system, on the whole, works rather better now than it used to in the 1960s when there was a terrible bottleneck and SRs waited until they were about 40 years old before being promoted. At least at that time they could 'drop off the ladder' and go into general practice, or emigrate to lands 'flowing with milk and honey' such as Canada or Australia. If the profession continues to expand faster than the number of posts within the NHS, we may see a return to those bad old days. Furthermore, in case this progress up the ranks until one is ultimately launched onto the placid waters of a consultantship has a cosy ring of inevitability, it must be stated that, in the keenly competitive specialties, this is far from being the case. There is a major bottleneck at the registrar to senior registrar transition, and a further one consisting of time-expired senior registrars, some of whom have to think of re-training in allied but less crowded specialized fields. The training years, then, are stimulating, challenging, rewarding, interesting, often even fun, but they are also years of long hours, intensive study, neurotic insecurity, and regular upheaval. Much of this period coincides with the phase of marriage and early parenthood, and this is perhaps why the marital track record of the profession is no better than that of the rest of society and is often claimed to be worse. Because of the uncertainty of securing a consultant appointment after this long and arduous struggle, the profession has from time to time attempted to match the numbers in the training grades with the anticipated number of consultant vacancies, with some success in a few specialties. The most recent of these attempts to alter the balance between seniors and juniors is much more radical than any of its predecessors, is likely to be implemented over the course of the next decade or so, and will profoundly affect the working lives of both.

Nowadays, a consultant is on average just over 37 years old at the time of his appointment. The RI, as I have indicated, has about 170 on its staff, and their specialties are listed in Table 2.2. Other countries such as France and the United States tend to have a steep hierarchy so that each department has a head: in the United Kingdom it is more of a plateau than a pyramid, and all consultants are, in theory, equal. They are not, of course, and there are various ways in which they are not. The most basic and mundane is the salary, and the scales for various grades of doctor (1987–88) are given in Table 2.3. From this, it can be seen that not only does the salary rise during the first few years in post, but also that there is a curious system of 'distinction' or 'merit' awards. The approximate proportion of consultants holding these awards is given in the table. The identity of the holders is highly confidential—it is not something you mention or put after your name. Recommendations are made after prolonged but discreet lobbying by a regional committee of some 18 consultants, all themselves award holders. Is the system fair? Many consultants, especially the younger ones, do not think so and are fairly strident in their views—and then, at a later stage in their careers, suddenly become mysteriously silent on the subject. All I can say, having served on the committee for a number of years and having chaired it once, is that it carries out its impossible task as conscientiously as it possibly can and considers every non-award holder in the region.

TABLE 2.2 Specialties of the RI consultant staff (1983)

Psychiatry	24
Anaesthetics	17
General medicine	12
Pathology	11
Radiology	9
Radiotherapy and cancer	9
General surgery	7
Obstetrics and gynaecology	7
Orthopaedics	6
Paediatrics	5
Ophthalmology	5
Bacteriology, virology	5
Neurology	4
Geriatrics	4
Cardiothoracic surgery	4
Rheumatology and rehabilitation	4
Dermatology, blood transfusion, biochemistry, ENT, cardiology, neurosurgery, chest diseases, dental surgery, urology	3 each
Immunology, plastic surgery, genito-urinary medicine (VD), haematology	2 each
Nuclear medicine, accident and emergency, nutrition	1 each

TABLE 2.3 Salaries of hospital doctors (1987/8)

Rank	Basic scale (£)	Addition (£) for nights on duty*		
		1 in 4	1 in 3	1 in 2
House officer	8810–9930	3205	4273	5697
Senior house officer	10 980–12 460	4008	5344	7126
Registrar	12 460–15 110	4218	5624	7499
Senior registrar	14 350–18 150	4387	5850	7800

		Addition for merit awards (% of consultants holding them)			
		C (22)	B (10)	A (3)	A+ (1)
Consultant	25 440–32 840	5790	13 000	22 750	29 550

* The figures are approximate and vary with the individual doctor and the individual post: doctors are charged for accommodation if married or if not compulsorily resident (e.g. first on call).

Furthermore, the fundamental qualification for an award is the provision of a fine service to the patients, and prolific research or brilliant lecturing count for little without that basic essential.

Another source of inequality is that a teaching hospital such as the RI has a number of university employed consultants. These are academic doctors, and there are five professors (medicine, surgery, pathology, obstetrics, psychiatry) and about 15 readers or senior lecturers with honorary NHS consultant status. An injustice is the fact that although they are paid rather better than non-medical academics, they are on a scale a little below the NHS rates, although they are eligible for distinction awards. (Conversely, NHS consultants do a considerable amount of teaching and hold honorary university titles as lecturers in the faculty of medicine.) Furthermore, the academics are not permitted to undertake private practice for personal gain and any proceeds from this source must be paid into the departmental research fund, research being a central activity to an academic but a somewhat peripheral one to most NHS doctors. Nevertheless, a professor enjoys a great deal of prestige and two of ours have knighthoods whereas the NHS can only boast a CBE or two. The professors write and lecture extensively and are in great demand at conferences all over the world. A part-time professor, it is said, is away part of the time, but a whole-time professor is away the whole time.

Finally, there is the question of private practice. The NHS was established in 1948 despite considerable misgivings by the profession, and among the concessions made by the minister of the day, Aneurin Bevan, in his eagerness to carry it through, were the system of merit awards and the right to carry out private practice in NHS hospitals. The profession withdrew its objections: 'I stuffed their mouths with gold', Bevan is reported to have claimed. Successive governments as well as the unions have proved so inimical towards private practice that it has become virtually separated from the NHS and the RI is only permitted a maximum of 16 private patients in its beds at any one time. Meanwhile, the private sector has expanded and flourished and a great deal of money which might have bolstered the dwindling coffers of the NHS has been diverted to the Nuffield Provincial Hospitals Trust which operates an excellent private hospital of 84 beds ('the gold mine') the other side of the city. This reflects a nation-wide trend, and although there are many situations in which the private sector currently has little to offer, it is an energetic and adaptable enterprise and there is no reason to suppose it will continue to accept these limitations. At present, there are three main contexts in which a subscription to a private medical insurance scheme is not particularly helpful. The first is the acute emergency—an accident on the motorway or a coronary at a dinner in one of the city's large hotels. The second is the realm of high technology – coronary artery bypass grafting (CABG), renal dialysis and transplantation, although in London such activities are increasingly on offer privately. The third is the protracted, multidisciplinary care of an elderly patient needing treatment for a number of common problems such as arthritis, heart failure, and stroke. Comfortable custodial care perhaps (although even this is not available on a long-term basis through many insurance policies), but active rehabilitation with a view to eventual discharge back home is seldom done well at the Nuffield. What the Nuffield does do well, it does superbly. It excels particularly in the field of elective surgery, carried out by the surgeon selected by the GP (and not his registrar), and carried out promptly and with sufficient notice and at a time convenient to the patient. Cataract extraction, plastic surgery, hysterectomy, hip replacement, hernia repair, and varicose vein surgery are examples which come to mind. Physicians at the RI have a comparatively thin time of it: some of us carry out a consultative practice at the Nuffield, but it is much less lucrative than surgery. It is ironic, in a society which generally places a higher value on cerebral activity than manual work, that a surgeon can easily perform a 20-minute operation and charge hundreds of pounds. The physician, who spends an hour taking a detailed history, performing a full examination and perhaps an ECG, and then comes up with some really exciting advice such as the desirability of losing 15 pounds in weight and stopping smoking, is thought to be overcharging if he submits a bill for much over £50. There is certainly one opthalmologist and one gynaecologist at the RI whose annual incomes are in excess of £150K—which makes the merit awards look rather paltry. Some orthopaedic surgeons are reputed to earn about £250K a year, but then a quarter of all hip replacements in the United Kingdom are done privately. Obviously, this is not possible while working whole time for the NHS—these consultants have maximum part-time (9/11) contracts with the NHS and drop 2/11 of their salaries and pension rights. They work very hard for the pickings: there is minimal resident medical staff at the Nuffield, so the consultant is often there at eight in the morning or nine at night. Is it satisfying?—some enjoy it, some not very much. For example, it is not possible to take a four-week holiday whereas a full-time consultant can: colleagues will quickly establish reputations with the GPs for greater availability—and availability is the name of the game: 'availability, affability, and ability'.

It should perhaps be mentioned that not all the specialties are equal. There is an unspoken pecking order, and in general, the more obviously glamorous fields of medical endeavour tend to be the more keenly sought after by entrants to the profession. Cardiology, heart surgery, neurology, and neurosurgery are perhaps among the most highly regarded specialties, with psychiatry, anaesthetics, and geriatrics towards the other end of the scale and the rest somewhere in the middle. One could think positively and put it the other way round – geriatric medicine and psychiatry offer the best career prospects.

What is it like being a teaching hospital consultant? It is a very demanding, very privileged existence. For one thing, the work is a constant source of fascination and satisfaction. For another, hospitals are exciting places to work in because one is surrounded by highly intelligent and highly motivated people. A consultant enjoys a very reasonable salary and a high degree of security. Finally, he leads a very varied life and is, to a remarkable degree, captain of his own destiny. I have a few beds in a small general hospital 18 miles away and also do a weekly out-patient clinic there. I do two ward rounds a week at the RI and visit my ward most other days, as well as having one out-patient clinic. That accounts for about half the week: then there is some teaching and a certain amount of administration, some late night committee meetings, papers and journals to read, lectures to prepare, some writing and a little research, and a whole collection of occasional commitments such as interviews, meetings in London in connection with professional associations, and various local or national clinical meetings. Many of these activities are at the choice of the individual consultant. A few become heavily involved in medical politics. Some rise to high office in one of the Royal Colleges. Others do a great deal of examining.

The public's image of the profession is that it is pompous, authoritarian, and conservative—perhaps with some justification. When you are in pain and frightened, you do not necessarily want your medical adviser to be a trendily-dressed swinger. You probably feel more reassured by a rather conservative figure who will tell you what he thinks is the matter with confidence and will discuss the action he proposes to take with conviction. The treatment he recommends will be based on a statistically sound, probably double blind, scientific study comparing it with other properly evaluated techniques: it will often have stood the test of time. Furthermore, it

will observe the first fundamental principle of medical practice—
primum non nocere. Do not expect the doctor, therefore, to be an
enthusiastic support of 'alternative' or 'complementary' medicine.
Does alternative medicine offer an alternative to insulin for diabetic
coma? Acupuncture, osteopathy, homeopathy, and similar art forms
offer poor substitutes for haemodialysis if your kidneys have stopped
working, or for intravenous diuretics if you have acute heart failure, or
antibiotics for septicaemia, or surgery for acute appendicitis. Nor
have they led to dramatic improvements to the general health
comparable to immunization against poliomyelitis, and they are
unlikely to do so until they achieve a solid scientific foundation.

3

Ministering angels:
The nurses

To be a doctor is widely regarded, with some justification, as desirable, enviable, and estimable: the sort of person you would like your son to become or your daughter to marry. To be a doctor is to be respected—but to be a nurse is to be loved. Compared with teachers, army officers, and the clergy, doctors do quite well in the popularity stakes. They are not in the same league as the nurses, who occupy a very special place in the public heart. Everyone knows they are overworked and underpaid. Everyone knows they are the people who really look after you when you are sick, while the doctors strut around pontificating in white-coated detachments. How far do the nurses deserve this public adulation? They certainly work irregular and often highly antisocial hours. When they are on duty, they certainly work very hard indeed and much of their work is exceedingly unpleasant. The actual hours worked, however, are far from excessive—37½ hours per week, a total which most doctors would regard as fairly modest. A great deal of the affection lavished on the nursing profession is undoubtedly accounted for by the fact that it is so overwhelmingly young and female. In 1981, there were nearly 400 000 nurses employed in the NHS, compared to 63 000 doctors including GPs. In terms of people, this figure would be considerably greater, but the NHS measures people in units called WTEs (whole-time equivalents), and a significant number of nurses are part-time. In our district, we employ just over 2500 of these WTEs (women of tireless energy?) but only 1600 of them work at the RI. The others include the Community nursing service (formerly the district nurses) and those who are employed at the psychiatric hospital, the long-term care geriatric hospitals, and the hospice. Those at the RI are scattered throughout the length and breadth of the establishment. They are to be found in large numbers on the wards. They are to be encountered in the out-patient clinics, the operating theatres, A&E, the X-ray department, the radiotherapy centre, the geriatric day hospital, and the labour rooms. In general, almost wherever you find patients, you will find nurses too, and they are also to be found away from the public gaze in the administration offices and the school of nursing.

The 400 000 nurses in the NHS account for between 40 and 45 per cent of the total NHS workforce and constitute the largest single group. The so-called ancillary workers (mainly concerned with hotel services such as laundry, catering, porters, domestics, and telephonists) come second with 167 000 or so immediately prior to privatization, which has taken a number of these services out of direct NHS employ. When studies involving large series of patients are described in the scientific literature, there is an overworked saw to the effect that for statistical purposes the subjects have to be 'broken down by age and sex'. Nurses do not readily submit to this treatment, but they can be broken down by grade. Of our 1600 nurses, half are trained, half are untrained: of those untrained, 245 are nursing auxiliaries who are not undergoing nurse training, and 475 are learners—that is, they are either student nurses who hope to become State Registered (SRN— now RGN, Registered General Nurse), or they are pupils who are aiming at the practical qualification of enrollment, State Enrolled Nurse (SEN). The learners are invariably youthful since they start training at 18, the auxiliaries are of varying ages, and the staff nurses and sisters start in their early twenties and continue into the thirties and forties and occasionally fifties. There are currently between 700 and 800 members of the nursing staff housed in hospital accommodation, although residence is not compulsory at any stage.

In recent years, the different species of nurse have become more readily recognizable since a degree of standardization of uniforms has been introduced throughout the country. The ward sister usually wears a dark blue uniform: at the other end of the scale, the auxiliaries wear yellow chequered with white. The others have pale blue dresses, again with a white check pattern, but it is here that difficulties arise due to differences between hospitals. An SEN usually wears a green belt and an SRN a blue one, but sometimes it is the hat which distinguishes the qualified nurse from the learner. Promotion to ward sister or the higher adminsitrative and managerial grades is only open to RGN qualified nurses, generally those who have also done their midwifery (if female) or mental nursing (if male). Girls hoping to become student nurses at the RI must have five reasonable 'O'-levels and are expected to take two 'A'-levels as well: candidates for SEN training only require CSEs. RGN applicants are selected for interview on the basis of their 'O'-level grades, and although only a minority are called for interview, about 80 per cent of those will be accepted.

Nation-wide, there is a very high wastage rate during training, about a third of those accepted falling by the wayside before qualifying and becoming registered. The salaries earned by nurses are really very ungenerous, particularly at the staff nurse and sister level when a great deal of responsibility goes with the job. A recent pay scale is given in Table 3.1.

TABLE 3.1 Salaries of nurses 1987–88

Nurse	Salary (£ p.a.)
Nursing auxiliary	4565–5855
Enrolled nurse (pupil)	4540–4735
Enrolled nurse (qualified)	6250–7750
Registered nurse (student)	4540–5170
Staff nurse (registered)	7040–8600
Ward sister	9000–12 000
District nursing officer	21 600–28 705

Note: these scales are increased by about a third for night duty and weekends worked: the London hospitals enjoy a special 'weighting'. The district nursing officer does *not* refer to the former 'district nurse' but to the most senior management role in the health district.

Deploying the staff is a major exercise since there are three shifts—7.30 a.m.–4.00 p.m., 1.00 p.m.–9.30 p.m., and 9.00 p.m.–8.00 a.m., to allow a degree of overlap between night and day staff. A ward of 24–28 patients will generally have five nurses doing the morning shift and four on for the afternoon and evening, so the individual may work two early shifts, two late shifts, and one morning (7.30 a.m.–noon) a week. The night staff will probably number two—either a staff nurse (RGN) and an auxiliary or a couple of SENs.

How do nurses spend their time? Anyone who has been in hospital will be familiar with many of their different tasks, but perhaps they converge to the greatest extent on the care of the high dependency patient. The medical wards usually contain patients who are semi-conscious, comatose, or paralysed. These patients need regular turning to prevent pressure sores; are likely to have catheters in their bladders and intravenous infusions to maintain; they require attention to eyes, mouth, and skin; they need periodic observation—pulse, blood pressure, respiration, temperature; if conscious, they need feeding, either by mouth or by nasogastric tube, and will certainly need reassuring, comforting, and positioning; and they are likely to need medication administered by one route or another.

Other patients need less constant attention but all are admitted and documented, weighed, and have routine procedures such as urine testing. Some come in filthy and need bathing at once, others need wounds or ulcers dressed or require enemas or suppositories. Getting the frail and aged up and washed, toiletted and dressed in the morning is itself a major undertaking. Then there are the drug rounds, which occupy two nurses, one of whom must be registered. There are meals, which on some wards are served by the domestic staff but on most, by the nurses. There are beds to be made. There are relatives to see, there are discharge preparations to be made, there is reporting to the next shift of nurses, there are doctors' rounds, there is inevitably the occasional death when the body must be cleaned and wrapped in a shroud—all these activities and many more, come within the overall sphere of nursing. It is perhaps not surprising that the Institute of Manpower Studies has suggested that the need for nurses is likely to grow so that by 1995 the projected number required will be over 550 000. In 1992, the Institute suggests, 35 000 students (some 45 per cent) will have to enter the profession to replace those leaving through marriage, pregnancy, or retirement, which is a much higher number than can be supplied by the current one in four of all girls leaving school with five O-levels and two A-levels who take up nursing. In fact, recruitment fell from 31 800 in 1982 to 22 000 in 1986, and 30 per cent of students give up before completing the course.

The high wastage rate and the likely shortfall in manpower is just one of the worries facing the profession, which is in the throes of upheaval, or perhaps a series of upheavals. Three major crises come to mind: the identity crisis, the turmoil over nurse education, and the turbulent wake of the introduction of general management.

From the brief description above, it might be thought that nurses undertook enough duties not performed by anyone else to assure them of their status as an independent profession. However, their own perception of their recognition in this capacity falls far short of their aspirations—or those of their leaders. To a large degree, it all boils down to the struggle to be free of the 'handmaiden of the doctor' image, the image of the doctor doing the clever, exciting, rewarding things (and being suitably rewarded), and then giving instructions to the nurses to do the routine, boring, smelly things (who then get miserably rewarded).

One response to this search for identity has been an attempt to define what is a nursing function and, rather more successfully, what is not. At one end of the range, a large number of rather menial clerical tasks such as filling in and filing forms, and taking telephone messages has been taken over by those most useful members of the team, the ward clerks. At the other end, there are endless demarcation disputes over tasks often assigned to the nurses by the doctors such as adding drugs to intravenous infusion bags and thereby effectively administering intravenous injections after the doctor has sited the needle. There are other minor procedures traditionally within the medical precinct, often carried out better by nurses, such as syringing wax from ears. The present moment is highly inopportune to declare these practices as non-nursing tasks rightfully falling to the doctors, since some nurses are currently mounting a campaign to become independent health-care practitioners who might become in most cases the first point of contact in the GP's surgery and who would undertake a great deal of the more routine clinical tasks including the diagnosis of common, minor ailments.

Another result of this struggle has been the emergence, largely from the Royal College of Nursing, that curious blend of trade union and institute of learning, of the 'nursing process'. This is a wind of change which encourages nurses to work in small teams each providing total care for their own group of patients rather than being 'task orientated' and going round the whole ward carrying out, for example, skin care. The nurses set their own goals for each patient quite independent of the aims of medical care, and indeed the nurse may assume the role of protecting the patient against the doctors. The introduction of the nursing process has made many of the doctors, particularly perhaps those with firmly entrenched attitudes, feel extremely threatened. In fact, much of it is very sensible and on a well-run ward there is no need for conflict because regular discussions take place between medical and nursing staff anyway. Rather more of a pity, perhaps, is the tendency to discard or reduce the medical input into nurse teaching.

It is, indeed, in the realm of education that the second great debate is taking place within the profession, largely fired by the looming shortage of trained nurses. A commission chaired by Dr (non-medical) Henry Judge reported on nursing education in 1985. It suggested that the high wastage is partly due to the current system whereby the students are employees of the health authorities and spend 65 per cent of their time carrying out much of the day-to-day work with intermittent periods of instruction in the schools of nursing which are situated within hospital complexes. Education would be removed to the campuses of higher education and the students would be supported by bursaries rather than salaries, and it is probable that the present two-tiered structure (registration and enrollment) would be replaced by a single qualification. In 1986, the UK Central Council for Nursing, Midwifery and Health Visiting (UKCC) made similar recommendations in the document 'Project 2000' and suggested that education should be broader, more community orientated, and slanted towards health rather than disease. Only 20 per cent of the students' time would be spent providing a service to the NHS. Again, there is much to recommend this approach, but again, there have been predictable howls of protest. A personal view would be that it might be a good idea, but that I do not wish to live through the years during which the change-over is taking place. In fact, it is already the case that some enlightened centres are offering four-year dual courses leading to both a university degree in any one of a number of subjects, and state registration. These courses attract, it is to be hoped, the future senior managers of the profession.

The whole concept of the manager is likely to evoke the third great shock-horror response among members of the senior nursing hierarchy. In the late-1960s another commission launched the Salmon report which introduced an entirely new career structure for nurses who did not fall by the wayside but who soldiered on after qualification and who devoted their working lives to the hospital service. Comfortable, familiar terms such as 'ward sister' and 'matron' were swept aside to make way for 'nursing officer (grade VII)' and 'senior nursing officer (grade VIII)' to the accompaniment of cries of derision from their medical colleagues. Whole new empires were built which, claimed the senior medical staff, downgraded the traditional supremacy of the ward sister and obliged her to desert the patients and their doctors for the desk and the committee room. During the next decade or more the NHS was reorganized twice and senior nurse management seemed to emerge more firmly embedded in the system on each occasion, although observers from the administrative and medical professions remained unenthusiastic about the senior nurses' expertise in the fundamental skills of man—or more often, woman—management. One unexpected phenomenon was the ascendancy of the male in a heavily female-dominated occupation, and a curious although entirely unsubstantiated personal impression would be that many of the senior posts came to be held by mentally trained nurses of Irish origin. This is not to imply any lack of administrative skills on grounds of race, sex, or training, but these skills certainly did not appear to be in abundant supply throughout the profession.

With the implementation of general management in 1985 and 1986 in the wake of the Griffiths report (Chapter 13), a Draconian dismantling of the whole top-heavy senior nursing structure took place with the inevitable consequences in terms of individual hardship. Posts vanished overnight, their holders had no jobs to fall back on, and large sectors of nursing organization were grasped by the new generation of managers from a wide variety of backgrounds both in and out of the NHS. It took the staff of the NHS a little while to wake up to what was going on. When it did, the response of the RCN was to launch a quarter of a million pound advertising campaign in the national press and the weekly magazines to try to convince a totally apathetic public that organizing nursing was a matter for the professionals and not for people who knew how to run a supermarket. At the time of writing, the issue is very much at the stage of 'watch this space' but it has to be said that morale in the profession is low. That is, in so far as the profession is represented by the desk-bound career nurse aged 40 plus. The problem with nurses is that such a high proportion of them are very young, female, worked off their feet, fascinated by their new experiences, and totally indifferent to the political strife in the upper echelons of the NHS or indeed to anything that may occur after registration.

Charlotte: 20 years old, second-year student nurse at a major London teaching hospital

I have been at St. Elsewhere's for a year and a bit. Eighteen of us started together, seventeen girls and one fellow. There are six intakes of about the same number each year. I suppose you could say we mainly come from a fairly middle-class background—my father is a GP in East Anglia—but we are a very mixed bunch and there are people from all walks of life. You need five O-levels and two A-levels although the grades and subjects do not matter much. I remember my interview very clearly. It lasted about half-an-hour and there were two senior nurses the other side of the desk, one being nice and the other asking a whole lot of very hostile questions like the 'good cop' and the 'bad cop' in a movie.

When you finally arrive it is very confusing at first because you have no idea who anyone is, but then you have a six weeks' introductory course before going on the wards. When you do start work in the hospital, you do eight or ten weeks on a ward and then go back to the nursing school before your next ten week attachment. Most of the lectures are given by the nurse tutors, but some are given by the doctors and they are usually better because they obviously know their subject so well. [She would say that, wouldn't she!—author.]

I have done two medical wards and one surgical as well as a childrens' ward, which I loved. I also did eight weeks in theatre, some of it as the scrub nurse and some in the anaesthetic department and some in the recovery room. My next duty is on A&E.

When you are on the ward you usually work from 7.30 a.m. to 4.30 or 5.0 p.m. three days a week, and 12.30 to 8.30 p.m. the other two days. You have two days off but it only works out at one weekend a month, except for while you are doing theatre because the weekends there are quiet. I am looking forward to cardiac surgery but not quite so much to psychiatry. We have a spell in maternity wing but only watch the births as observers because the student midwives are helping out during labour.

When you do a medical or a surgical ward you do night duty for a couple of weeks—one week on, 8.45 p.m. to 8.0 a.m. every night, one week off. There was just me and a staff nurse who was a permanent night nurse. At first it was quite fun but after a while the life becomes rather unnatural.

Theatre sister is a real battleaxe and so are one or two of the others, but most of them are really helpful. Nothing really prepared me for my first death which was during my first medical ward. You have to wash the body, dress it in a shroud, put the teeth in and close the eyes. Staff nurse had the worst job which was telephoning the relatives. Then there are all the belongings to collect and list.

You can move out of hospital accommodation as soon as you like. I found a flat after nine months or so—I much prefer it to living so much on top of my work. The hospital rooms are too small, anyway. My social life does not really revolve around the medical students. We are always invited to their parties, and some of them are quite good. They hold balls from time to time, and they are really good. But the medical students are an even more mixed bunch than we are.

I have heard that nurse education may be moved into the colleges and away from hospital, but I think most of it is really too practical for that to work properly. But I would prefer to have a better theoretical background, because the patients often do not understand what the doctor tells them and then they ask us. I do not think anyone is specially worried about AIDS, but we are very careful to put needles straight into the sharps box and not back into their sheathes. I haven't really thought about the future very much, but I think it would be fun to work abroad for a bit.

Penny: 36 years old, Director of Nurse Education

I have only been in post here for a couple of months but I was doing the same job down in Cornwall beforehand. You could say that I am the most powerful and senior nurse here, although I am concerned with tomorrow's patients rather than today's. I qualified dually, children and SRN, and after being a ward sister I became a representative for an appliance manufacturing company. That was quite an eye-opener!

It did not take me long to find out that I have got a tough job on my hands. The English National Board (ENB) visited a few months ago and they have made some pretty severe criticisms. And the consultants and the Health Authority were never even told! The attitude is all wrong—just because it is the RI they seem to think they have a God-given right to train nurses. Some of the wards do not even try to teach them. I will have to take the students and pupils off those wards and put in more trained staff and auxiliaries instead, but I am afraid there will be howls of anguish.

Yes, I do think that a system of education in which the learners are supernumerary is the right way forward. I have already started a dialogue with the university, so something might happen early next century. It works well in other countries. After all, why should we be the only profession in the NHS which is trained on the job? But I agree that the changeover period will have to be brilliantly planned if it is not going to be a total shambles.

Maureen, 37 years old, ward sister on 'my' ward

I qualified at the RI and have worked there almost ever since. I am responsible for a 26–bed general medical ward and I suppose that my job could be described as a combination of head of household, hostess, nurse, and manager. Most of my life is spent running around organizing the other nurses and their off-duty times and helping them and teaching them. I try to get around the patients every day and, instead of standing with arms folded like the doctors, I sit on the side of the bed and I think that is much less threatening. I also enjoy doing the medicine round because that way I also get to see all the patients. But I suppose only about a third of my time is spent in direct patient contact.

Ordering supplies takes three or four hours a week, and I am responsible for that although I sometimes delegate it to the others. One of the most important items I order are food supplies. For instance we use 4 lbs of tea and 10 lbs of sugar a week, as well as cereals and fruit squashes and some 10 loaves of bread over and above what comes up from the kitchen. We order drugs to maintain our stock of two or three hundred which we always keep. That includes enemas and skin creams, of course. And then there are stores—such as 450 cardboard bedpan liners a week, 350 urinals, plasters, and sputum pots. There is crockery to replace breakages. There are CSSD supplies—syringes, catheters, sterile dressings, drip giving sets. Cleaning and similar products are mainly brought to me by the cleaning firm, but I order 200 toilet rolls a fortnight and 50 bars of soap. And finally there are other minor items such as endless plastic bags.

I have to make sure that repairs are carried out—electrical, plumbing, carpentry, and it is really just like home because it helps enormously to be friendly with the craftsmen and offer them a cup of tea. And there is an endless stream of people to greet, like patients and ambulance crews and relatives and doctors from other wards and senior nurse managers and administrators and dieticians and therapists and chiropodists and the chaplains and the voluntary workers and endless porters and so on, and so on.

It takes a week to get to know each new house physician and to decide if he is going to be sensible and conscientious and good to the patients and nice to work with. Most of the nurses quite enjoy doing practical procedures for the doctors like syringing ears and taking blood samples, if they are confident enough to do so, but there seems to be a tendency to restrict the tasks that nurses are allowed to perform. We like to do anything we can to help, and at the other end of the scale, if there is a shortage of clerks or porters or domestics, guess who does the chores!

I think that one of the changes is that sisters are less autocratic nowadays. We tend to believe in consensus management. I know that it is not in line with the new fashion in the health service, and I am very worried about the new managers. If I have no senior nurse above me, I will have to run the ward budget, and I will have to hire and fire the staff, and go to an agency if I am short of staff, and how on earth can I do all that?

I would dearly love to see student nurses spend more time in the classroom instead of being used as pairs of hands, but certainly not all their time. They would arrive on the wards registered and thinking they knew it all but really knowing nothing. It is a practical training, when all is said and done. We have a girl with a degree in nursing from another city, but she is not as good as my staff nurse who has just qualified from the RI.

4

Shop window:
Accident and emergency, out-patients

Hospitals are often rather unfairly depicted as ivory towers which protect the rarified atmosphere of scientific medicine within from the importunate demands of an obstinately suffering public without. The barriers which separate the two are in fact breached daily by the hoards of maimed and halt who throng the A&E department and the out-patient clinics. The knights in armour who breach those defences are mounted on the gleaming white chargers with streaming red and blue banners provided by the ambulance service. The ambulances are much in evidence on our roads, especially on the streets immediately surrounding the RI. For many people suddenly brought face to face with disaster, they bring relief, reassurance, resuscitation, and rapid transportation from the scene of the tragedy.

The ambulance service is organized along the lines of the old county boundaries, and there are stations in most towns of any consequence. Our service therefore covers three health districts, and we have a number of scattered stations of which the largest is housed in a hangar-like building in the south-eastern corner of the RI site. The county ambulance service possesses 74 vehicles of which 30 are emergency or 'front-line' ambulances, and they have an impressive range of standard equipment (Table 4.1). The remainder are more concerned with the routine 'bussing' of patients to and from out-patient clinics, day hospitals, day surgery, and non-urgent admission and discharge. The clear distinction between these two activities was eventually established only in 1986 and was in most people's views, long overdue. It is anticipated that there will now be a two-tier service, and it is to be hoped that the planned conveyance of the infirm to and from their place of treatment will no longer be subject to unpredictable disruption by the overriding needs of the steady supply of the injured who are scraped up off the motorways. The County service now undertakes well in excess of 1000 patient-journeys on each working day (Table 4.2). This includes the enormous assistance it

TABLE 4.1 Standard equipment for emergency ambulances

Minimum equipment
First aid kit
Blankets
Vomit bowls
Incontinence pads
Bag and mask—selection of airways
Carrying chair (if vehicle has stretchers) (none if seats only)
Additional equipment
Additional first aid kits and blankets
Stretcher poles and canvasses
PneuPac IPPV Resus/fixed-flow respirator set
Analgesic equipment—self-administered
Suction equipment—electric and manual
Selection of splintage including traction
Burns sheets
Maternity packs
Scoop stretcher
i.v. fluids—cannula and giving sets (doctors use)
Intubation kit (not all vehicles, due by 1987)
Monitor/defibrillator (not all vehicles, due by 1987)
Fixed 'F' size free-flow oxygen
Personal intubation kit
Intravenous infusion kit and fluids
Monitor/defibrillator (portable)
Drug administration kit
Medical antishock trousers (all by 1987/88)

TABLE 4.2 The ambulance service: number of journeys undertaken (1983 and 1985)

Year	1983	1985
Emergency calls (County)	11 250	12 300
Urgent calls (County)	7800	10 150
Routine patient journeys by ambulance (County)	101 300	101 150
Total patient journeys by ambulance (County)	*120 350*	*123 600*
Hospital car service journeys (County)	128 250	152 450
Total patient journeys (County)	*248 600*	*276 050*
District emergency calls	4850	5350
District urgent calls	3600	4300
District emergency plus urgent	8450	9650

receives from the hospital car service which reimburses some 100 private car owners at the rate of 16p or 20p a mile for ferrying patients back and forth who cannot cope with public transport, have no one to drive them, are unable to afford a taxi, but only require minimal assistance from one person. As a doctor, it is often very hard to submit an honest request for transport on medical grounds in cases where such a large proportion of the need is really social.

At the RI a staff of 26 trained ambulancemen man the front-line crews and they work three shifts; the early shift from 7 a.m. to 3 p.m. when there are usually seven crews on; the late shift; and night, when there are three crews on duty. The basic pay in 1986 is £165 weekly, and the cost of a journey works out at about £3 per mile. The job entails a fair amount of inactivity, but when the action comes, it comes fast. The calls are divided into three priorities, of which the top is 999. There are about 1000 of these per month but in London the number runs into many hundreds a day. They mainly originate from members of the public, often at the roadside, unlike the other categories of call, which are made by GPs. An 'urgent' request is made by the GP from the patient's home, and requires a response from the ambulance service within two hours, and a 'red' call is again initiated by the GP who indicates that immediate transfer to hospital is necessary. While responding to an urgent call, the crew may be notified by radio of a 999 call on their route and will be diverted to administer what life-saving measures they can until the vehicle assigned to that call arrives. A large number of the emergency calls are to road accidents and the majority of the others are for people who have collapsed due to heart attacks or strokes. The heart attacks constitute a particularly worrying group because so many of them are salvageable ('hearts too good to die'), yet the incidence of fatal electrical disturbances of heart rate and rhythm is at its highest within minutes of the event of coronary artery thrombosis. For this reason, some pioneering centres have trained ambulance personnel in the diagnosis of the exact nature of the disturbance from the electro-cardiogram and the administration of appropriate intravenous drugs or electrical DC shock. This high-tech intervention can pay dividends in terms of lives saved but incorporates the usual practical difficulties of maintaining a permanently available, fully equipped vehicle with a fully trained crew, dedicated to this particular task. Since human beings have unfortunate characteristics of requiring time off to sleep, meet their families, and go on holiday, it is probably necessary to have a pool of five crews highly skilled in cardio-pulmonary resuscitation (CPR) to ensure that one is available round the clock throughout the year. Which brings us back to the constantly recurring theme which the ambulance service has become all too familiar with in recent years. The reorganization of the service into its two separate functions already mentioned was widely predicted to bring about significant savings. It therefore came as no surprise that what actually followed its implementation in February 1986 was an overspend of £400K during the course of the following financial year. We are currently waiting to learn how the public is going to cope with the ensuing drastic curtailment of conveying patients too infirm to travel by public transport and too poor to come by taxi, for essential out-patient treatment.

The first port of call for the victim of a road traffic accident (RTA) rushed to hospital by a blue-flashing siren-shrieking ambulance in full cry is the A&E department. It is also the first port of call for many local citizens of all shapes and sizes making their much less dramatic entrances with an enormous range of accidents, injuries, and illnesses, some grave, some trivial, some gory, some clean. A&E has a fine sweeping approach and an imposing portico to allow the ambulances to decelerate and unload their damaged cargoes under cover. The 'walking wounded' have a far less impressive doorway from the main approach road, and then have to register with the clerk at the desk and sit in the waiting room glancing through tatty 18-month-old copies of the Sunday colour supplements, while trying vainly to catch the eye of any passing nurse or doctor in order to emphasize the urgency of their plight. Inside, A&E is a more-or-less open-plan football pitch of a place with two main areas. One is Admissions, where medical, surgical, gynaecological, or paediatric emergencies alerted by their GPs are examined by the on-call SHOs and registrars and undergo initial urgent investigations and treatment and are either allowed home or found a bed. The endless tales of patients kept hanging about for hours quite often misrepresent time spent just as usefully as it would be on the ward. There are, it is true, occasions during the winter months when the hospital seems to be bursting at the seams and yet a never-ending stream of wheezing, coughing, gasping old people with chest infections and heart failure are wheeled in by the ambulance crews. The bed-state was accurate at midnight the previous night, but the ward clerks may not have notified all deaths and discharges to the head of the bed bureau, who may have to undertake a patrol of the wards in order to identify recently vacated beds, and then consult with ward sisters and eye surgeons who, rightly, wish to admit patients who have already waited far too long for their cataracts to be extracted. Meanwhile, downstairs there is the nightmare of stacking 15 sick people with accompanying relatives in Admissions with only two nurses to attend to them and to the newcomers.

A&E proper has two cubicalized reception areas, a comprehensively equipped resuscitation room with three tables, a 'dirty' theatre, a recovery area, a plaster room, and two X-ray rooms. The current number of patients attending is over 42 000 a year—or the number of attendances, to be more accurate, since 3000 are re-attendances to have sutures removed, etc. Just over a fifth are children, and trauma accounts for two-thirds of these. All human life—and death—is there. About 500 deaths occur annually, either brought in dead (BID) or dying on arrival despite attempted resuscitation. Many of these are RTA victims, others will have sustained a massive myocardial infarct (see Chapter 7) or stroke. There are 50 000–100 000 sudden deaths in Britain a year, most of whom have coronary artery disease. Other grave emergencies include overdoses (50 per month and 14 per cent of medical admissions), acute abdominal catastrophies including bleeding from the gut, and various accidents sustained elsewhere than on the roads. The less serious cases are legion—elderly people falling and sustaining a fractured wrist or hip or nothing except being rather shaken; children with foreign bodies in ears, nose, or (not necessarily children) eyes; dog bites (man's best friend inflicts 209 000 bites a year requiring treatment in England and Wales); sports injuries; burns and scalds; lacerations caused by fights or by domestic accidents; raging toothache due to dental abscess; the sudden and painful inability of an elderly man to pass urine. If it happens at home, the doctor is called, but if it happens in a public place or at work, the chances are that it is a 999 call if dramatic, and self-referral to A&E if fairly minor. It is axiomatic in medicine that no one is simply a case of such and such a disease, but a unique individual with a unique problem, and nowhere is this more true than in A&E which witnesses a steady trickle of one-off predicaments which no one has ever previously managed to land themselves in, to tax the ingenuity of the staff. For example, one of the local sculptors decided to create a mask of his own face and prevailed upon his assistant to cover his face with plaster to form a cast which would serve as a mould. Unfortunately, he became inseparably attached to the plaster due, no doubt, to his exuberant beard and duly presented himself for hammer and chisel treatment, still breathing through the straw which the assistant had thoughtfully inserted before applying the plaster.

The staff of the department are savers of lives, restorers of order out of chaos, assessors of priority, bouncers of those abusing the system. They are also, increasingly, themselves victims of violent assaults from drugged or drunk youths. There are three sisters and 16 staff nurses, of whom five are on at any one time. There are six SHOs, most of whom are training to be surgeons or GPs—an excellent training is obtained during a six-month spell in A&E. The casualty officers work in shifts, two, three, or four on at any one time, except nights (midnight-8 a.m.) when there is only one. The shifts are 8 a.m. to 4 p.m., 10 a.m. to 8 p.m. and 4 p.m. to midnight except weekends which are divided into 12-hour shifts. There is one day off a week and alternate weekends: the nocturnal casualty officer goes to bed in the on-call room. The job is often memorable, can seriously interfere with one's social life, and is emphatically not an easy job. It is, in these respects, like most other SHO posts. The casualty officer can, and often does, seek help from the appropriate specialty who will send a registrar or senior registrar. There is an SR in the department who is training to become a consultant. In overall administrative charge, deploying his troops, handling police and press enquiries, sometimes rolling up his sleeves and entering the fray himself, is the energetic and able consultant who is the Director of our Accident Service. He knows almost as much about the working of the RI as anybody in it, so who better to co-ordinate the hospital's response to a 'major incident'?

Every major hospital has to have a plan of action in preparation for the eventuality that a train or aeroplane disaster occurs in the vicinity or that an explosion devastates a public meeting or a department store in the city. In such circumstances, the police are in overall charge of rescue operations and their control room will inform the Fire Service, the Ambulance Service and the hospital switchboard. The switchboard notifies 15 or so key people, several duty registrars and consultants from the appropriate specialties together with a number of others (accident, orthopaedics, surgery, neurosurgery, anaesthetics, haematology, medicine, nursing, administration, mortuary technician), and other medical and nursing staff report to A&E apart from theatre staff who make sure the operating theatres are in a state of preparedness. The co-ordinating Medical Officer in overall charge at the hospital is the Director of the Accident Service, while the police retain command at the scene of the incident. Senior medical and nursing personnel are responsible for clearing beds to make way for the flood of casualties, and the transfusion laboratory is alerted to the imminent arrival of batches of blood samples for cross matching. The mortuary staff is also instructed to expect an influx of victims. The first GP on the scene of the disaster becomes the 'Incident MO' and he is in close contact with the Co-ordinating MO and is responsible for establishing a medical control post and deciding whether to call out a Hospital Mobile Surgical Team and, if necessary, a blood transfusion service refrigeration van. The former consists of a surgeon, an anaesthetist, and three nurses together with the equipment required to render life-saving assistance such as assisted ventilation or emergency surgery: the latter carries blood, plasma, transfusion sets, and a haematologist and will support the mobile team. The administration and medical records staff will document the patients on arrival at the hospital as well as handling relatives, effecting liaison with police, ambulance service and Incident and Co-ordinating MOs, and diverting minor cases to nearby 'second-line' hospitals. It all sounds like a military operation, and military operations have a reputation for proceeding like clockwork on paper but becoming an utter shambles in the heat of the battle. One day it is inevitable that our major incident procedure will be put to the test. Meanwhile, the Mobile Surgical Team is required to turn out from time to time to salvage lives on a more modest scale. For example, a farmer in his late thirties overturned his tractor in a remote ditch, crushing his leg which held him pinned to the ground. The team carried out an amputation on the spot, and despite this appalling cost he has made an excellent recovery and was soon able to return to work.

Although for many, their point of delivery to the RI and their introduction to it is through A&E, for others it is through the portals of the out-patient department. There are 12 clinic suites on two floors each accommodating from two to four doctors and they all have a common spacious entrance hall and a little cafeteria. Along the length of this concourse opposite the entrance is a long desk with six windows where the medical records staff process the documentation of each patient and direct them to the appropriate clinic, rather like the check-in desks at an airport. The postal or telelphoned request from the GP for an appointment for his patient is passed to the girl who deals with the clinics for the consultant specified. She will arrange the appointment, depending on the degree of urgency indicated, by feeding whatever information she has into the master index. If the hospital number is available, the index can be accessed at once and the computer terminal will display the patient's treatment periods, consultants' names, wards, and discharge dates so that locating the notes should be easy. Otherwise, it is a question of asking the master index for details of all the John Smiths and hoping that the date of birth, address, or even the GP's name will enable the correct one to be identified. The computer will also offer the clerk a number of appointment times and she will notify the patient of the one she has selected. If a follow-up appointment is required, the patient presents the clerk with a slip stating how many weeks ahead the doctor wants to see him again, and the clerk again feeds this information into the computer.

Many specialties carry out an increasing proportion of their patient care on an out-patient basis. These include skin and eyes, dental surgery, diabetes, rheumatology, and fractures. The fracture clinic, in particular, is invariably awash with the never-ebbing tide of life's mishaps and tends to present rather a conveyor-belt impression. Every weekday afternoon it receives the victims of RTAs, icy pavements, rugger tackles, and hysterical horses. The patients have been manipulated and plastered in A&E or the orthopaedic ward, and come to the clinic to be X-rayed, reviewed, and perhaps to have their casts changed for lighter ones or, better still, removed altogether. Plaster of Paris remains very much alive and well in 1987 and there is only one manufacturer who supplies it to all NHS hospitals. Some units have changed to newer, lighter materials which usually have a slightly grubby brownish appearance as well as costing a great deal more. At the RI we now incorporate some glass fibre into below-knee casts which make them lighter and increase the cost from £3 to £20 each. We have five two-man fracture clinics weekly and between 40 and 90 patients each time, of whom 80 per cent will require plasters. In 1985, over 4200 new cases were seen in the fracture clinics and there were almost 13 400 attendances altogether.

Skin clinics take place every available session, in other words every weekday morning and afternoon. The consultant and one or two assistants see 10–20 new patients and perhaps a total of 60 each time, and carry out a few minor operations to remove or sample unsightly excrescences.

The diabetologist estimates that he has 12 000 or 15 000 insulin-dependent diabetics on his books, and 80 attend each clinic but are shared among five doctors. Four or six new diabetics turn up each week, and others will be seen in general medical or geriatric clinics. Perhaps 10 patients attend the pregnant diabetic clinic. All the diabetics will have their eyes examined annually to detect the abnormal blood vessels now dealt with so effectively by laser treatment.

This is another out-patient procedure, but it is performed by the ophthalmologists in their highly specialized out-patient suite. They too have continuous clinics in which seven doctors see up to 120 patients a day. Their instruments take up a great deal of space (and money: the laser cost £50K), so the place tends to become rather congested. In all the big clinics, sheer numbers tend to get in the way of smooth organization and transport difficulties cause further disruption. It is all too common for patients to be kept waiting an hour or so, which often makes the first encounter with the hospital's shop window a not particularly happy one.

5

Mainstream medicine and
its branches

The title of this chapter is unashamedly biased since those of us in general, internal, hospital-based medicine consider it to be central to all medical activity. We are more highly specialized than general practitioners but do not engage in such distasteful activities as surgical operations. Most of us practice a sub-specialty in addition to general medicine. Some of us, having undertaken training in the various medical specialties and having successfully presented ourselves for the examination for membership of the Royal College of Physicians (Chapter 3), have become exclusively sub-specialists or super-specialists, depending on one's viewpoint. For instance, few neurologists practice any general medicine, nor do the dermatologists, but some cardiologists and chest physicians do and so do a few geriatricians and many gastro-enterologists and most endocrinologists and nephrologists. The true 'general physician' is almost extinct and the vast majority of consultants in general medicine appointed nowadays are expected to have a specialized field of expertise as well as participating in general medical 'takes'. What all this boils down to is that the organization of the medical specialties in British hospitals is a kind of chaos without anarchy, so that nobody claims exclusive rights over their own domain and everybody poaches to a greater or lesser extent on everyone else's territory. For example, the geriatricians and the 'general physicians' look after more arthritis than the rheumatologists, more patients with strokes that the neurologists, more patients with heart failure than the cardiologists, and more patients with pneumonia than the chest physicians. Conversely, it is probable that geriatricians only see a minority of all medical patients over the age of 65. A great deal of cross-referral goes on. Most patients with heart failure respond quite quickly to the standard treatment given by a house physician straight out of medical school. Some do not, and some patients have different and more difficult cardiac conditions, and then the team in charge of the patient will request the cardiologist to come and see him and advise whether further tests are required, perhaps involving a transfer of care to the department of cardiology for further investigations and treatment.

Medical students spend more time attached to general medical and general surgical firms than they spend grazing in the other fields of medical activity, and those are the main core subjects in their examinations: those, and pathology, on which everything else is based. When they qualify, it is in general medicine and general surgery that they do their two six-month 'house jobs'. These, then, are the two giants of hospital practice, and of the two—well, who needs to know about surgery except the surgeons?

At the RI we have four medical firms each with two consultants and each owning a 28-bed mixed-sex ward. A couple of the firms each have an additional consultant from the rarified realms of academe who look after the occasional patient with his special illness, although the professor of medicine himself is one of the mainstream physicians. Each firm has about two-thirds of a senior registrar, a registrar, a senior house officer, and two house physicians. The firm also has the nursing staff and the secretary: but the physio- and occupational therapists and social workers are shared out among the medical block rather than owing their allegiance to any one firm.

The vast majority of the patients on the ward arrive as emergencies via A&E or via the admissions unit, which is really an offshoot of A&E, where the GPs are invited to send patients they feel are acutely sick and who they have discussed over the phone with the registrar. He will go and see the patient there, examine him, decide whether he needs admission, and if so, find an appropriate bed, send off blood tests and arrange preliminary X-rays *en route* to the ward. This procedure saves a great deal of time, even though it may still seem to involve endless waiting around if you are on the receiving end. Eventually, probably about two hours after the ambulance delivered you at the entrance of A&E, you arrive on the ward, where the ward clerk or nurse carries out further documentation and where the house physician descends on you as soon as he or she is free to do so. The house physician then repeats all the questions your GP and subsequently the registrar have already asked, only in much greater detail and followed by a much more comprehensive examination, for the fomer two were merely taking decisions whereas the house physician's notes are the definitive account of the clinical picture. Then, when you think you are going to receive some actual treatment, it may be meal-time or wash-time or temperature-taking, or urine-testing time. In case all of this sounds rather an anticlimax after the drama of being 'rushed' to hospital with sirens screaming and blue lamps flashing, it must of course be added that if the condition is a life-threatening one, treatment will obviously have already been started: heroin or morphine and a diuretic and oxygen for acute heart-failure by the GP; intravenous antibiotics for a nasty pneumonia by the registrar in admissions; an i.v. line for a bleeding ulcer by the casualty officer.

As far as possible, the on-take firm absorbs this daily tide of ailing humanity and will have tried to discharge as many patients as practicable in preparation for going on-take, in order to make beds available on its own ward. By tradition, the only admissions electively farmed out to other wards are long-standing patients of the firms concerned. The case mix of patients therefore reflects the current pattern of acute medical emergencies more than it does the special interests of the consultants: unlike the highly-specialized departments and the regional specialties, it is uncommon for patients to be transferred in from hospitals in other districts to access the refined skills of the teaching hospital consultants. There is a slow trickle of cold, or elective patients who have been seen in the out-patient clinic, whose flavour clearly mirrors the tastes of the consultants. A considerable amount of medicine is practised according to what are variously termed 'flow charts' or 'algorithms'. For example: a late-middle-aged patient, is tired, lethargic, found to be anaemic. Are the blood cells small, pale (iron-deficient), reasonably normal (chronic disease), or large (vitamin B_{12} or folic acid deficiency, among others). If iron deficient, is the diet inadequate or does the patient habitually take aspirin or anti-arthritic drugs, which may cause oozing from the stomach? Or is he bleeding due to an ulcer, or due to a cancer? If so, is the cancer upper gastro-intestinal or lower? Questions are asked, the abdomen examined, the stools investigated for traces of blood, and depending on the balance of probabilities, either the gullet and stomach or the colon are investigated by means of radiology or endoscopy.

Most of the initial 'work-ups' of the patients on a medical ward will have been arranged at house physician and registrar level. They will have been on the receiving end as the emergencies came in, moribund from blood loss or diabetic coma, during the small hours of the morning, they will have called the surgeons for one patient, sat up half the night checking blood sugar results for another. They will have the satisfaction of presenting a viable, sentient, relatively normal being to the consultant when he does his round. They will, by then, have exercised a considerable degree of autonomy in deciding what investigations to order: perhaps a head scan for someone who has started to have fits; perhaps a venogram for someone with a painful, swollen leg. They will also have carried out such practical tasks as seem necessary. Blood transfusion for the bleeders; a lumbar puncture to obtain a specimen of the clear, colourless fluid in which the brain and spinal cord are bathed, for the severe sudden onset headaches, to see if there is blood or pus: a needle into the space between lung and chest wall where fluid has accumulated, for the severely breathless, to see if it contains bacteria or malignant cells. In addition, there are the X-rays, the endless blood tests, and the electrocardiograms. All the results are gathered, scrutinized, filed, and mentally pigeon-holed for the ward round.

It is fondly imagined by the consultant that his ward round is the focal point of the week. Sister is usually there, the patients are there, the visitors are gently discouraged from being there, all the junior doctors are there, and even the X-rays are supposed to be there. The ward round still goes on because no one has yet really thought of anything much better. Too often, it goes on *and* on. Many of the most important decisions have already been taken because they had to be. Theoretically, all the major policy decisions are left to the ward round—which often simply means, can this patient go home how, please? There are long discussions over patients whose initial crisis is over but who still pose problems of diagnosis or treatment. The cast is typically assembled in attitudes related to their roles. The patients, anxiously trying to divine what the muttered phrases portend. Sister, fidgetty and bored, thinking of all the other things she has to do. House physician, fearful what errors of omission may come to light and apprehensive how many hours of work today's decisions will entail. Registrar and senior registrar, vying for points for thinking up further possible diagnoses. The chief, wishing they would not and wondering what all these new syndromes, investigations, bugs, and drugs are anyway. The consultant goes round perhaps twice a week. The others do their rounds daily. It is no longer true, I hope, that doctors will pause and converse at the foot of a bed without even addressing its occupant, a practice which has rightly been deplored by various groups which protect the patients' interests. After introductions, the house physician will recount the history and describe what heart murmurs or breath sounds or lumps and bumps he has found: the others will then listen and probe more or less in order of seniority, and will agree or disagree, the revealed truth being encapsulated in the consultant's opinion of the findings. Then there are X-rays and ECGs to look at and the results of blood counts, biochemical tests, and bacteriology. Finally, the various treatment options have to be considered and the corporate advice discussed with the patient. The whole exercise is rather like a roving committee, with the consultant (or, if he is away, the senior registrar) as its chairman and the houseman as the hon. sec. furiously scribbling minutes to remind himself of the various tasks the committee has allocated him. A ward of 28 patients takes two to three hours, and if most of them are new, it is rather hard work. On my ward, we then have tea. It is a working tea, especially for the houseman, and the social worker, physiotherapist, and occupational therapist (OT) join us. We discuss each patient again, only this time, it is not so much the serum gamma-glutamyl transpeptidase level as the home circumstances, the support available, the ability for self-care that is the main thrust of the discussion. Some physicians are very impatient with 'social problems' and regard patients for whom the hospital has done all it can but who have resolutely refused to become well enough to go home, or who have no home to go to, as 'bed-blockers'. These are likely to be aged and impoverished, and suffering from long-term diseases such as strokes. It is true that at the RI we may have up to a ward full of these unfortunate souls, and that they may cause difficulties in admitting the acutely sick. It is not true that they cost a fortune—they use fewer resources than fresh emergencies and actually do their bit towards keeping costs down.

The physiotherapists, unlike nurses, do not receive a salary while training but a grant from the DHSS, also, they spend their three years training in school, although their school is also within the grounds of the RI. To enter our school, you need three 'A'-levels with fair grades, and there is an annual intake of 20 for the three-year course. The students do not enjoy university vacations, but holidays of four–eight weeks a year, similar to workers in the NHS. Once qualified, they contribute enormously to patient care, shifting sticky bronchial secretions, building up wasted muscles, enabling stroke victims to regain the skills of standing and walking. There are 30 of them at the RI and they treat large numbers of out-patients as well as those on the wards, the annual number of treatments totalling an amazing 38 000.

We have 20 occupational therapists, who are also closely involved in rehabilitation and in enabling the stricken to relearn the basic skills of self-care after a devastating illness or accident and who will also advise concerning any gadgetry that may make life easier for the disabled. Like the nurses, the therapists are struggling to emerge from medical domination. Co-operation and relationships are excellent, but the struggle is there, just below the surface. Like the nurses, they feel that their qualifications should be based on a university degree. The two professions, it must be said, lack political muscle—not because of their overwhelming female preponderance, partly because of the relative youth of most of their members—but mainly because of their relatively small numbers.

As mentioned earlier, most physicians have a special interest which indicates a particular field of expertise and probably the acquisition of certain technical skills. Every general hospital will have a gastro-enterologist trained in upper gastro-intestinal endoscopy. He will do one or two sessions a week and will examine both in-patients and out-patients, both his own patients and those referred from other consultants in the hospital. There remains a degree of controversy concerning the respective merits of endoscopy and radiology in the investigation of suspected ulcers or cancers of the gullet, stomach, and duodenum, but endoscopy has certainly become a very routine procedure during the past 15 years. At least one of our experts prefers to do the examination on a patient who has not had any preparation other than fasting, and without using any sedation at all, and he encourages the patient to go back to work afterwards. Perhaps eight patients are dealt with during the course of a morning's session and we have several endoscopists who do some 1200 a year between them. The procedure has been made possible by the development of fibre-optics, so that the instrument, about a metre and a half long and the thickness of a man's little finger, can be steered round corners and yet the light source still illuminates from the tip, and the eye of the observer accompanies the tip in its journey into the interior. In addition, there is a narrow tube down which the operator threads a flexible biopsy forceps so that small bites can be taken from any suspicious looking site and sent for microscopic examination. The steering knob directs the tip whichever way it is desired to look. Since the value of the device is some £10K, a guard is placed between the patient's teeth to stop him damaging it. The only other preparation is a spray of local anaesthetic to the throat, and the patient lies on his side and the procedure is over within five or ten, rather uncomfortable, but far from agonizing, minutes. The endoscope goes down the oesophagus, with its uneven, undulating walls: into the stomach, where the lining is thrown into folds like furrows in a field: through a dark hole at the far end, and on into the duodenum where the folds run right around the wall. The mucous membrane lining the various passages of the body should be a soft glistening pink: not an angry red, and not studded with small bleeding points. Although usually used for diagnostic purposes, it is sometimes possible to use the endoscope for treatment such as the dilatation of an oesophageal stricture or the injection of oesophageal varicose veins to prevent a torrential haemorrhage. The much more difficult, time-consuming, and unpleasant procedure of colonoscopy is essentially similar from the point of view of the abnormalities the examiner is seeking: only about 200 are performed a year.

The other super-specialists each have their own stock-in-trade. The chest physician of my youth had accumulated a vast experience of the many and varied manifestations of tuberculosis. He has been replaced by another wielder of the serpentine endoscope, this time to look at the bronchial tree and to take samples of cells and of the secretions. Bronchoscopy is usually performed through the nose and the instrument is very much slimmer than the gastroscope. The nose, throat, and vocal cords are sprayed with local anaesthetic, the instrument is lubricated and passed down the trachea and manoeuvred into the area of interest as shown on the X-ray. The bronchial tree has a ribbed or corrugated appearance due to rings of cartilage and the branchings tend to be very acute. A permanent record of their appearance can be obtained by the injection of contrast down the endoscope followed by a series of X-rays. The work of the chest physicians is spatially close to that of the cardiologists, but discussion of the latter, like the neurologists, properly belongs in Chapter 8. The chest physician of today can also investigate structural abnormalities of the lung by drilling out small portions to scrutinize under the microscope. However, much of his work is concerned with the function of the lung, with how well it shifts air in and out and how efficiently gas exchange takes place between the air and the blood, and for this purpose he has a laboratory which carries out a series of 'lung function tests'.

Although contagious diseases remain major scourges of the developing world, they play a fairly minor role in a modern British hospital. The infectious diseases ward (ID) has 12 individual cubicles where the quarantined status of the occupant is emphasized by the disposable gowns and gloves worn by all visiting staff and by the air conditioning which provides 15 air changes every hour. Most of the unfortunate inmates isolated in these lonely and rather cold cells are suffering from surprizingly mundane illnesses. Acute diarrhoea is assumed to be infective until proved otherwise, hepatitis (jaundice) is infectious, and shingles can transmit chicken pox to those who have not already had it. There is a steady trickle of tuberculosis, but this is now regarded as constituting a very low public health risk almost as soon as chemotherapy has been started. Children with measles, mumps, chicken pox, and whooping cough are virtually always looked after at home, but a few come in when the social back-ground makes this impossible. The occasional case of poliomyelitis and the annual crop of travellers who slipped up on their antimalarial tablets are treated in ID largely, I have always suspected, as a punishment since the public is over-whelmingly immunized against the former and there is no risk of person-to-person transmission of the latter. That leaves the dreaded MRSA—described vividly in the local paper under the banner headline 'Killer Bug Hits City Hospital'. The initials stand for methicillin-resistant *Staphylococcus aureus*, an unpleasant bacterial strain which not only causes severe surgical wound infections, pneumonias, septicaemias, and abscesses but is immune to virtually all the conventional antibiotics. This particular organism crops up fairly regularly, particularly among the sickest patients, and those afflicted are transferred to ID. Sometimes it is not identified in time to prevent a minor outbreak, for instance in the intensive therapy unit, which then has to be closed until it can be properly cleaned with a solution of phenol. If the ITU is closed much of the surgical activity of the RI is severely restricted.

General physicians, during recent years, have to a considerable extent demolished their reputation for inactivity by developing the specialized technical skills we have considered, and have thereby become almost extinct. There remains one activity which physicians and geriatricians use more than any other in order to treat their patients, and that is prescribing. The traditional medical approach to a sick individual is to take the history, conduct a physical examination, draw up a list of likely possibilities, arrange the necessary special tests, and thereby arrive at a diagnosis and formulate a plan of treatment. The treatment strategy may incorporate several elements: a blood transfusion for anaemia; advice about smoking and exercise; asking the dietician to explain the dietary requirements of his condition to the patient, especially, for example, in the case of diabetics; physiotherapy for locomotor problems affecting joints or muscles. However, most patients on medical or geriatric wards will receive a course of drug treatment or may indeed be started on long-term medication or have their previous drug regime modified. The apparently simple process of receiving a medicine involves three independent professions—the doctor who prescribes it on the individual patient's prescription chart, the nurse who administers the pill or the injection, and, unseen by the patient, the pharmacist who dispenses it.

The pharmacy at the RI is divided into three main sections, those for in-patients and out-patients being on the ground floor, and the central pharmacy being in the basement. There are eight staff pharmacists including the chiefs, and eight basic grade (recently qualified) pharmacists. It is an all graduate profession, the degree awarded by the university being either a Batchelor of Science or a Batchelor of Pharmacy. This is followed by a pre-registration year of which half is likely to be spent in a retail pharmacy (a high street chemist's shop) and half either in hospital or in industry, before achieving the professional qualification of Membership of the Pharmaceutical Society (MPS). Once again there is the same story of difficulties both in recruitment to the hospital service, and retention of existing staff, due to unfavourable salary comparisons with retail pharmacists. In 1986, a basic grade pharmacist in the NHS starts on an annual salary of £7014, but those in private retail can expect to earn £11K or £12K on registration. There are, in addition to the professional staff, 11 technicians who do much of the routine dispensing and some 40 clerical and secretarial personnel. Apart from the supplies and works department, the pharmacy is the only purchasing unit in the hospital, but it also still carries out a certain amount of its own manufacturing of items such as disinfectants, lemon syrup, mouth lubricants, and liquorice and peppermint water, as well as some sterile preparations of eye drops and intravenous fluids which are produced by gowned and masked technicians in what is probably the most sterile room in the hospital. In this room, the bacteriologists leave little dishes of jelly lying around, which are impregnated with delicious broths to tempt any passing germs to express their appreciation in the only way they know how—explosive multiplication. Any deterioration in the sterility of the environment would thus be reflected in tell-tale circular creamy colonies of bacteria.

The pharmacy dispenses about 350 in-patient prescriptions and 200 out-patient prescriptions a day. It holds some 2700 items which are mainly reputable pharmaceutical products of one sort or another, but which also include antiseptics for cleansing wounds or floors, acetone to remove nail varnish, bags of electrolyte solution for intravenous infusion, and whiskey. Time was, within living memory, when hospital dispensaries manufactured a number of pills and tablets. Today the shelves are stocked with a bewildering variety of attractively packaged products of the giant multinationals, from diuretics for heart failure to anti-inflammatory agents for arthritis to antibiotics and antidepressants, and a host of other categories of medicine. Most are made available in several forms, and after the initial patent has expired, by several companies, so that recognizing a tablet can be difficult. There are tablets, sugar-coated pills, capsules, ointments, suppositories, injections, and sustained-release preparations. The keen eye will discern the manufacturers' representatives on the prowl around the hospital corridors, exploiting the uneasy interface between industry and the professions. They often hunt in pairs, increasingly frequently consisting of a reasonably presentable male science graduate and a stunningly presentable ex-nurse or female science graduate. They are not in uniform and therefore are not staff, but they are on business and therefore are not visitors or patients. They visit the pharmacy and they lie in wait for the doctors. They also, it must be said, promote a very large number of medical meetings which otherwise could not take place because there are no other sources of funds to pay visiting speakers their travel expenses, let alone a fee, or to provide modest sustenance to replace the lunch or dinner that attending doctors will forego. The hospital consultant may not write many prescriptions, but his teaching will influence the prescribing habits of future consultants and GPs. He is wooed by the industry in a highly acceptable way when a research registrar or even a working registrar is funded by 'soft money' from this source. He is courted in a less acceptable way when he and his wife are taken for skiing holidays with all expenses paid. The latter experience is a form of corruption which most of my colleagues read of in the newspapers but have yet to experience. Nevertheless, it remains a rather unpalatable fact that the drug industry in this country spends £2.5K a year per doctor on promotion. Of this expenditure, 80 per cent is on GPs and amounts to £5K per GP.

The other link between hospital staff and the manufacturer is in the realm of testing new drugs. The company will do the necessary animal work and the studies on healthy volunteers. Eventually, a new drug has to be tested on patients and this is where the grey reputation of the academic physician arises. Patients have to be used as guinea pigs, because otherwise the outlook for future sufferers of incurable and fatal disorders (for example, senile dementia) is bleak indeed. So a promising new drug, safely taken by healthy human subjects, is given to a group of patients who have agreed to participate. A tablet or capsule identical in appearance but containing a totally harmless substance (the placebo) is given to another group of consenting patients with the same disorder. Patient preference, adverse effects, and any measurable benefit from the drug are recorded and the active and dummy tablets switched over. Neither patient nor doctor know which is the real course of treatment and which is the placebo: the only person who does is the statistician who ultimately analyses the results. Sometimes the outcome is a profitable launch for the manufacturer, a prestigious publication for the medical staff conducting this laborious study, some 'slush funds' into the departmental research account, and, most importantly, an improved treatment for future patients. More often, perhaps, the tests reveal nothing of any value.

Perhaps it is time to swim against the current of mainstream medicine briefly and explore shortly some of its tributaries. One of the larger of these at the RI, is geriatric medicine. In some hospitals the geriatricians share wards with the other physicians and simply take the most aged patients. At the RI, they have their own territory, three wards in all, and the decision as to whether a patient in his or her seventies goes to general medicine or geriatrics depends mainly on who has a bed, but also on the diagnosis—more strokes go to geriatrics, more diabetic crises go to general medicine, more hypothermias go to geriatrics—following reasonably amicable discussions between the duty registrars concerned. When there is a shortage of beds, disputes begin. The geriatricians are hoist by the petard of their name. It simply means the medicine of old age, but the media have corrupted it by association with the negative image with which they have tarnished old age itself. The result has been to produce a pejorative term which is constantly misused: there is no such being as 'a geriatric'. The geriatricians handle a great deal of heart disease, a great deal of chest disease—a great deal of disease. They do much acute work, and 70 per cent of their admissions go back home again, although quite a few die. They are strong on rehabilitation, but for the 5 or 10 per cent of their admissions who survive, but fail to regain independence, there are the peripheral geriatric hospitals where they are transferred for long-term nursing under the overall supervision of one of the consultants. These hospitals have no resident doctors but use the local GPs for day-to-day care and have no diagnostic facilities, so they are run comparatively cheaply. Comparisons can be misleading, however, and the cost per patient per week is about £230, thus anyone who survives a couple of years has cost the taxpayer £22 360, which is considerably more expensive than a heart transplant. However, in spite of extreme age and frailty, survival for two years in a long-term ward is common because the standard of care behind the forbidding exterior of the old workhouse is very high.

One of the activities of the RI which has engendered a strikingly clubby, almost family atmosphere among the patients is the renal unit. It occupies rather indifferent premises towards the periphery of the site because it is totally reliant on car-parking facilities since the patients take themselves to and from treatment. These are people whose kidneys have become so damaged by one of a number of disease processes that they are unable to eliminate toxic waste products (or even, for that matter, simple chemicals such as potassium or water) as fast as they accumulate. Some of these diseases are fairly gradual. At first, the damaged kidney works satisfactorily unless stressed: then it starts to fail and affects the general health: then it virtually ceases to function, which is not compatible with life. Sometimes this sequence occurs quite abruptly and although these patients usually recover, sometimes they do not. We have, at the RI, between 150 and 200 patients with 'end-stage renal failure' to look after, from the city and a little beyond and from quite a few of the neighbouring districts. There is a range of treatment options, including allowing the patient to die which might be the most humane course if the kidney disease process affected other systems too in a relentlessly progressive manner. In most cases, however, it is only the kidneys which are severely diseased, and some other means must be found of performing their work. The most highly favoured is renal transplantation, but life must be preserved and health restored while waiting for a donor, and this is achieved by chronic haemodialysis—the 'artificial kidney'. Acute haemodialysis is the term used when use of the artificial kidney is likely to be short-lived and self-limiting, because the kidneys have temporarily ceased functioning as a complication of acute renal disease or of a serious accident or of some infectious illness, particularly if there has been a catastrophic fall in blood pressure. Under these circumstances, the kidneys often recover quite quickly if the patient is kept in good general condition and in reasonable fluid and chemical balance. Sometimes it takes a little longer and the extra time is bought by haemodialysis to correct the blood chemistry, if it is going dangerously haywire. Sometimes they do not recover at all, so the patient is effectively without any kidneys and faces the same plight as people with chronic progressive renal disease.

Chronic renal patients can usually be maintained in reasonable health by fairly simple measures for a period which may amount to several months or years after diagnosis: and this means many years into the illness, for the symptoms are so subtle that it is highly unlikely that chronic renal failure will be diagnosed until it is so far advanced that anything up to 70 per cent of the kidney tissue has been destroyed. Gradually the tiny filtration units in the kidneys shut down until the fine tuning of the regulatory mechanisms become over-stretched and the physical and chemical constants of the blood vary outside the narrow limits which are normally so scrupulously observed. The patient then has too much water on board, or too little water on board, or the blood is too acidic, or contains too much potassium (which can stop the heart), or there are too many circulating waste products, and anaemia develops—eventually the unfortunate victim starts feeling extremely rotten. There are various strategies for coping, for a while. Plenty to drink, perhaps, to wash the poisons through. A low protein diet, to retard the accumulation of nitrogenous waste products. However, 'end-stage' renal failure finally ensues. The chronic dialysis programme is for those who effectively have no viable kidney tissue left. It is carried out in a converted ward with 15 beds and the patients arrive in two shifts some days, three shifts other days. Each patient has two sessions a week lasting from three and a half to six hours. They all have indwelling vascular access—in other words, tubes leading from an artery to a vein, usually in the forearm, which they disconnect from each other and link up to the machine, often with very little help from the nursing staff. If the shunt blocks or becomes infected, it may have to be re-sited elsewhere — and there is a limit to the number of sites available. However, the shunt often lasts a long time, and one of our patients is now in his twelfth year with the same one. The patients arrive from a radius of 50 miles around by bicycle, bus, or car and greet each other and the staff with varying degrees of cordiality: it is striking how well some of them look, how unwell others. What the treatment does offer is reasonable freedom from dietary restriction except for fruit and other items high in potassium.

The machines are really simple pumps which augment the efforts of the patient's heart to provide a head of pressure of 150 mmHg. The blood is pumped through a cylindrical object almost a foot (0.3m) long and perhaps three inches (7.5 cm) or so in diameter: this contains

11 000 cuprophane (similar to cellophane) tubes each 11 microns (thousandths of a millimetre) across which are bathed in the dialysate fluid, some five litres being used each time. The blood passes down these exceedingly fine tubes, and the nitrogenous waste products of protein metabolism pass out into the dialysate solution together with excess potassium and, in effect, the two fluids reach an equilibrium which restores the chemical composition of the plasma to normality. The filter costs about £7 and is generally discarded after a single use. The current age range of the chronic haemodialysis patients is 12–75 years: as more patients enter the programme, others leave it—by death or by transplantation.

Renal transplantation requires a donor kidney of correct blood group and tissue type, as well as a rather formidable regime of drugs to suppress the recipient's immune system which would otherwise reject the foreign organ. Some of these drugs (usually prednisolone and azathioprine) are continued indefinitely in smallish doses, but they still tend to cause stunting of growth in children. It is nevertheless a superb operation for a significant number of patients, more than a third of them surviving five years with the first transplant and more than a quarter for ten years. One of our patients is alive and well 20 years post-transplant, and the youngest survivor received his transplant at the age of two. If the donor organ is rejected the procedure can be repeated: one patient received six transplants, although the circumstances were rather exceptional. In 1984, 1443 kidney transplants were performed in the United Kingdom and there were estimated to be 3500 patients living with functioning grafts. We do rather over 70 kidney transplants a year, and sometimes the grafted kidney works at once and sometimes the patient needs a week or two on dialysis before the implanted organ picks up and takes over.

For those for whom the chances of a successful operation have been discarded, there are two alternatives to permanent twice-weekly visits to the club. We have almost 70 patients whose intelligence and domestic stability have permitted the installation of pumps in their own homes where, helped by their families, they carry out 'do-it-yourself' dialysis. They are the out-stations of the haemodialysis unit, and have telephone access to our technician as well as regular checks by physician and nurse. Their 'groceries'—the dialysate bags and the filters—are also supplied by us. The other programme which we have instituted quite recently for patients with end-stage renal disease is chronic ambulatory peritoneal dialysis, or CAPD. In this technique a tube is inserted from the exterior into the abdominal cavity and the membrane lining the cavity is used as the filter between dialysate and blood. Two litres of fluid are run into the abdomen and left for two to three hours before being run out and replaced with fresh solution. This exchange is performed by the patient four times a day. This technique is growing in popularity, rather surprisingly, and our first dozen pioneer patients are keeping well and finding it quite acceptable. Their supplies of 'groceries' for the week are rather bulky—56 litres a week—and there is a risk of infection, so they have a hot-line to headquarters. The longest recorded duration for a single CAPD intra-abdominal catheter is an exceptional 11 years.

The 'club' is presided over by the consultant nephrologist, who is also a general 'on-take' physician. He selects the patients for the various forms of management and is responsible for their education and that of their families. He shares a longer and more intimate participation in their illness than almost any other consultant. It is difficult to remain detached when a long hoped-for transplant is successful: or when, as occasionally happens, it works for a while and then fails and the disappointed recipient receives the commiserations of his fellow members as he reluctantly resumes his regular visits to the club.

Another highly specialized service is clinical haematology, which at the RI, is really a euphemism for the regional leukaemia service. They are divided between two territories since their patients under 14 years of age are looked after in the childrens' wards and their adults occupy 15 or 20 beds in the medical block. There is, in fact, a wide age scatter with this group of diseases, just as there is a wide scatter of their degree of severity. Those with the more malignant varieties of leukaemia are admitted for an initial period of about five weeks when they will receive a very rigorous course of cytotoxic chemotherapy with multiple toxic drugs given in very high doses monitored by repeated examinations of aspirated specimens of bone marrow. The object of this treatment is to poison the malignant cell lines in the marrow, and while this is going on the patient needs to be kept alive. The unit therefore uses a great deal of blood and its products since the patients are likely to be anaemic or to bleed due to a lack of platelets or to develop virulent infections due to inadequate white cells and suppressed immunity. If one of the patients should be found to harbour a particularly nasty invading organism, he will be barrier nursed in a single room where he can only be visited by masked, gloved, and gowned figures who wash carefully after examining him and dispose of his cutlery, crockery, and excreta using special precautions. The rooms are reasonably pleasant and receive filtered air to minimize the chances of this type of infection. There was, until recently, a fashion for 'reversed barrier nursing' because of the susceptibility of these subjects to infections, and some centres had isolation chambers in which no contact was permitted with the outside world. Staff would gain access to the patient by remaining sealed inside an enormous sleeve of polythene entering the room from the exterior, and the sleeve had its own sleeves and gloves so that blood could be taken using the syringes, needles, and bottles which were already in the isolation chamber. These were recovered, like the meal trays, from the double-doored 'out' hatch, while the meals were delivered after irradiation through the 'in' hatch. This type of precaution may be revived if we embark upon a marrow transplantation programme in which the patient's marrow is destroyed, together with all the malignant cells, by massive irradiation and then replaced by intravenous injections either of his own bone marrow specially treated to eliminate malignant cells or of marrow from matched and preferably related donors. This finds its way back to the bones and starts manufacturing red cells, white cells, and platelets, but meanwhile the patient is exceedingly vulnerable to any passing bacteria.

The number of adult patients with acute leukaemia who survive five years from diagnosis is now about 25 or 30 per cent, but a far higher number, perhaps 75 per cent, achieve a worthwhile remission lasting a year or 18 months in which the disease has effectively become dormant. Forty per cent of those may actually be cured of the disease. The RI receives one or two new adult acute leukaemics a month referred from the region, and perhaps the same number of children.

Clinical haematology also undertakes plasmapheresis, a technique for separating off the elements of the blood to eliminate immune complexes or abnormal proteins or leukaemic white cells and replacing the blood with normal white cells and plasma and the patient's own red cells. The replacement products are obtained from the patient's family or from volunteers from the local military, who are blood-grouped and tested for virus infections. The subject (or donor of white cells), semi-recumbent in front of an apparatus, which looks as if it has come out of an amusement arcade, is bled from a vein in one arm while the machine centrifuges off the plasma or white cells and replaces the healthy plasma into a vein in the other arm. This may be done once a month for five days for up to about two hours, and is therefore a fairly costly exercise in terms of staff time. The equipment is not particularly cheap, either, and the overdue replacement of our old 'banger', a first-generation instrument some 15 years old, will cost us £20K or £30K.

A little further exploration brings us to what can, perhaps, without causing offence, be called the backwaters of medicine: skin and VD, or to use the official titles, dermatology and genito-urinary medicine. The skin doctors have an image among their colleagues of not knowing what the rash is caused by, but of giving it a long latin name to give the impression that they do, and treating it with the same topical corticosteroid ointment that anyone else would use anyway. They see a large number of patients with internal diseases with external manifestations; they see a large number of fungal problems; they are deluged with leg ulcers; and they spend a great deal of time giving advice on other peoples' wards. They have a ward of their own too, where leg ulcers which have defied decades of changing fashions applied by district nurses, get put to bed and heal up magically— often to break down again within a few months of being sent home. If you have a more abstruse skin problem, you get photographed and biopsied and then you get treated and then you get photographed and biopsied again. This rather subjective image of dermatology is partly founded on envy: no night calls, few emergencies, and plenty of private practice.

Venereology is an exclusively out-patient specialty and it differs from the other medical specialties in that it is open to the public to take themselves there without a GP's letter of referral. The department also has its own case records separate from the patients' hospital folder, to preserve the strictest confidentiality, and seldom writes reports to the patients' own doctors. The service is based on a lone consultant who is backed up by two or three GPs who do a few sessions each. Like the cancer doctors and the geriatricians, and psychiatrists, he is at high risk of being asked 'don't you find it depressing?'. He is energetic, able, and enthusiastic and clearly finds overworked and suppurating genitals a source of endless fascination. His department deals with 4000 new cases annually, of which nowadays very few are the traditional venereal diseases of syphilis and gonorrhoea. Non-gonococcal urethritis is not only the commonest sexually transmitted disease (STD)—it is the second commonest infectious disease in the country after the common cold. This, and the viral diseases such as herpes and warts, comprise the bulk of the caseload. Much of the work is tracing contacts and a very high proportion of these are homosexual: straight sex remains a comparatively low-risk activity between non-promiscuous partners. Homosexuals and drug-takers are groups with a particularly high risk of being infected by AIDS (although female partners are also vulnerable), and the ethical dictate is that if you have a very sick patient you do whatever blood test may contribute to the diagnosis without asking permission, but if you have a high-risk patient with some totally unrelated problem, then you should seek permission before asking the laboratory to look for the AIDS virus. A positive test will be followed by counselling. The strictest confidentiality must be preserved at all times, because positive status renders the carrier a social and occupational pariah. Therefore, the fact that a patient is an AIDS carrier is not stamped all over the hospital notes, although some health service staff feel that it should be, for their own protection. The label on the notes merely states 'Infection risk from blood', which might equally indicate the hepatitis virus. It is also permissible to package blood samples from such people in special envelopes similarly labelled so the laboratory staff know that they require particularly careful handling. If these patients are admitted for any reason, it is to the infectious diseases ward where they can be effectively isolated and where staff visiting them will be gowned, gloved, masked, and wear protective spectacles. At the time of writing it appears that AIDS is likely to become a major problem in the United Kingdom although there are hopes that the newer antiviral drugs are going to prove effective against it. It has certainly had a profound impact on medical training in the United States. A physician recently described its effect on the training of an internist (general physician) in San Francisco. An intern (houseman) it seems, is likely to have one or two sufferers under his care at any one time, and by the time he completes his residency training, he will have seen more cases of AIDS-related pneumonia than ordinary pneumococcal pneumonia and more cases of AIDS-related cancer than cancer of the breast. Medical technology may be constantly changing, but so is disease.

The medical specialties include the bread and butter of the local practice as well as some of the more exotic cases from far and wide. The rheumatologist, for example, is never short of custom and beavers away dispensing the latest anti-inflammatory drugs and arranging physiotherapy and referrals for joint surgery, but seldom requires recourse to admission. The vast majority of the general in-patient work consists of emergency admissions, hence we have little control over our expanding caseload. Our remit is to take what the local GPs send us, turn it round and send it back home again as fast as we can to make way for the next occupant of the bed. We feel we are under too much pressure to give the best deal to the patients, many of whom would benefit from convalescence. From the vantage point of the mid-1980s it is remarkable to recall that we enjoyed convalescence facilities until the mid-1970s—a luxury that is almost unthinkable in the setting of today's service.

6

Blood and guts:
Surgery

When they come to fetch you, they wheel you away from the ward in your own bed. You are wearing one of those ludicrous gowns open down the back which makes it easier to remove when you are unconscious. You are lying flat on your back, which gives you a new and mysterious perspective of the passing scene as the porters push you along the corridor, take you up to the top floor in the bed lift, and then along another corridor to the theatre receiving room which is rather like another ward. From your horizontal position it is difficult to see much of what is going on, but the 'pre-med' has made you so woozy and carefree that you do not mind any of these indignities. Indeed, you are concentrating far more on swapping brilliant jokes with the porters than on your surroundings. The effects of the 'pre-med', the anaesthetic, and the pain-relieving drugs used for the first few days post-operatively combine to blur the memories of an experience most people would rather forget anyway. So although many of us sooner or later enter an operating theatre suite, very few retain any mental picture of it beyond the curious world of glass and great round brilliant overhead lamps, populated by unidentifiable ghostly green-clad figures wearing caps and masks, so regularly portrayed on our television screens. It is a world which its regular inhabitants regard with affectionate familiarity but where the occasional visitor never really feels at home.

The dictators who strut the corridors of the suite are the consultant surgeons. At the RI we have a number of highly specialized surgeons fulfilling our extra-territorial commitments, but first and foremost we have the usual surgical staff to be found at any DGH. There are seven general surgeons, most of whose work lies within the abdominal cavity and is concerned with the gut and its appendages. Two of them have in addition special expertise in vascular surgery and deal with the veins and arteries of the legs and abdomen. There are six orthopaedic surgeons: orthopaedics really means 'straight children' because the specialty originally dealt with deformed and crippled children, but it is now concerned with trauma, and with bone and joint surgery. We have three urologists whose province embraces kidneys, bladder, and prostate and the various tubes which connect them to each other and the outside world. We have seven gynaecologists whose specialty is divided into women with disease of the pelvic reproductive organs, and the delivery of babies which is conducted over in the maternity department. There are also the very specialized surgeons, the otorhinolaryngologists who much prefer the title ENT (ears, nose and throat) and the ophthalmologists (eyes): three of the former, five of the latter.

The main theatre suite at the RI is quite impressive and consists of 10 theatres in a straight line together with their annexes. However, there are other theatres scattered around the complex: two in the neurosciences block, two in maternity, the two 'dirty' theatres next to the infectious diseases ward, the day-case theatre, and one each in the A&E, cardiothoracic, and radiotherapy departments. The principal suite is almost at the top of the main ward block: almost, but not quite, because a considerable quantity of expensive machinery has to be housed above the theatres in order to keep them running. From the outside, it is easy to see the great grids which provide the air inlets lining this topmost layer of plant which is the preserve of the mechanics and engineers. This air is filtered, humidified, warmed, and pumped down into the theatres which thus have a slightly higher pressure than that prevailing outside. As you pass them, you can see that each has a flap to the corridor which is lifted by the soft current of air passing through. Usually, the air in an operating theatre changes about 22 to 28 times in an hour. The work of the orthopaedic surgeons is even more liable to the ravages of infection than that of the other surgical specialties, so one of their theatres was equipped with a laminar airflow unit at a cost of £30K seven or eight years ago. This is a grid forming the whole of one wall of the theatre which further filters the air and directs it in a carefully shaped flow pattern over the table, increasing the hourly air changes to 300. It hums gently to itself and you can just feel a very slight draught: all of the theatre staff ensure that they stand downwind from the operation field as far as possible to minimize any potential bacterial contamination. All this filtration ensures a permanent supply of clean air. Constant humidification at 55 per cent prevents the possible hazard of sparks of static, and a temperature adjustable between 18 °C and 24 °C provides a comfortable working environment.

The theatres and their adjoining rooms are arranged linearly

behind a long corridor which is, in turn, just behind the patient
reception area. This is the clean corridor which means that you have
to change before you enter it. Behind the theatres again is the dirty
corridor, equally long and straight, and this is where the used
instruments, towels, swabs, and all the detritus of a surgical operation
are despatched after each case. The next port of call for the patient,
whom we left in the reception area, is the anaesthetic room which is
situated at the entrance to each operating room, where the anaesthetist
lies in wait with his reassuring small-talk and his unreassuring battery
of needles, ampoules, bags of saline, and his positively alarming
trolley of airways, bags, and gases. The theatre porters wheel the bed
down the clean corridor and lift the patient onto an operating table in
the anaesthetic room where he is anaesthetized and then trundled into
theatre. Occasionally the patient will be anaesthetized in his bed
before being transferred onto the table, particularly if he has, for
example, a broken leg which makes manhandling uncomfortable.
After the operation, the patient is moved to the 'patient out' area and
transferred back onto his bed. He is then taken to the recovery ward
which is opposite the receiving room where he is supervised by
nursing staff while he recovers consciousness. When they are satisfied
that he is fit to undertake the journey, perhaps 20–40 minutes after
leaving theatre, he embarks on the long haul down to the ward. In
some of the more major cases, or in particularly high-risk patients, the
anaesthetist may insist on checking the patient's condition himself
before allowing him to leave the theatre suite.

   The surgical staff go in through the senior medical staff changing
room. If you are male, you strip to underpants and socks, and if
female, I suppose to some sort of equivalent in an adjacent room. You
put on a pair of clean blue pyjamas with short sleeves, and your short
white boots, and a cap: this outfit entitles you to enter the clean
corridor and find your way to your theatre. Down a narrow corridor
and into the scrub room: put on mask, scrub hands, wrists, forearms,
under mixer tap with elbow-handles using pink disinfectant for five
minutes: split open paper pack, put on sterile gown unfolding it in
such a way that outside surface of gown touches nothing: sterile
talcum over hands, letting excess fall direct to floor: select partly
folded back glove, only touching inside: slip on one glove, use that
hand to pick up other and put it on without gloved hand touching
ungloved hand: tuck sleeves of gown into gloves without touching
wrists with gloved fingers: and stand waiting for unscrubbed staff
member to do the ties at the back of your gown. You may then enter

the theatre, where your sterile gloves may only touch the sterile
instruments passed to you by the scrub nurse—or the (generally
sterile) insides of the patient. Between each case you scrub all over
again and put on fresh gown and gloves. So who are the *dramatis
personae*? For a moderate operation—a gall bladder or a breast, for
instance—there might be: the patient; the anaesthetist (unscrubbed),
at the head end; the surgeon (consultant, senior registrar, or in less
major cases, registrar); his assistant (registrar or house officer); the
scrub nurse (sister or staff nurse); her runner (unscrubbed); operating
department assistant (ODA, there are 22 of them); perhaps another
ODA, auxiliary or student nurse (unscrubbed); perhaps a medical
student or two (unscrubbed); if it is an orthopaedic case, perhaps a
radiographer; and, if it is a showbiz spectacular such as a major
transplant, a bevy of visiting surgeons from overseas (unscrubbed).

Theatre staff are available round the clock for emergencies, but the
routine office-hours procedure is for each theatre to have a booked list
each morning and afternoon of the working week. Same session each
week, same surgical team, same anaesthetist, same scrub nurse. Each
surgical team might have two, three, or even four regular lists a week.
The scrub nurse has a major responsibility for presiding over the
proceedings and ensuring their smooth running. Her first task is to
wheel a trolley round the local 'supermarket'. This is the TSSU
(theatre sterile supply unit) which occupies a room the size of a
badminton court half-way along the suite between the clean and dirty
corridors. At any one time in the working day there might be a dozen
ancillary workers, all in theatre clothing, receiving the dirty instruments and towels from the dirty end, putting them into the washing-
up machine, taking them out of the drying machine, and wrapping
them up in sealed packets for re-use. These packages are then
sterilized for 40 minutes by steam at a pressure of 32 lbs per square
inch and a temperature of 135°C in one of the three autoclaves. All
three were, until very recently, showing distinct signs of wear and tear
after 10 years of constant use and there was something very
incongruous in the three plastic bowls standing under them to catch
the drips of rusty water, in the midst of all this sterility. They have
recently, at last, been replaced, at a cost of £20K–£25K—running the
theatres uses up a great deal of money. After they are taken out of the
autoclave, the packages are put on shelves in a store at the clean end
of TSSU. Some shelves are orthopaedic, some gynaecological, some
general: and some packs are marked THR (total hip replacement)
and some are marked 'anterior resection' and some are marked T and

A. So the scrub nurse collects everything she needs for the list, and stacks them in her instrument room, and unpacks them all and lays them out on her trolley before each case.

The TSSU, it may be mentioned here, is a sub-station of CSSD (central sterile supplies department), which prepares all the packages used for dressings, catheterization, deliveries, and innumerable everyday nursing and medical procedures, as well as tremendous numbers of theatre packs. The scale of the operation may be judged by its clients. It supplies all the wards, the day-case theatre, maternity, 12 health centres, and the community nurses as well as raising some much-needed revenue by servicing a private dental clinic and a local acupuncturist as well as helping out the Nuffield when it runs a little low. Perhaps it is not too surprising, therefore, to learn that the 25 members of its staff turned out three and a half million packs last year, most of which were rapidly used. Once sterile, they stay sterile (unless the theatres are invaded by the dreaded Pharaoh's ants which get everywhere and which live in warm air ducts: I asked the difference between a Pharoah's ant and the common-or-garden variety and was merely told 'Pharaoh's ants are red, they bite, and they reach the parts other ants cannot reach'. Luckily, we have escaped such an invasion—so far). CSSD uses a bank of four autoclaves similar to those in TSSU, together with another which operates at 70 °C with or without formaldehyde but for a longer duration to treat non-heat-resistant items such as fibre-optic endo-scopes. CSSD receives the dirty packs, washes the contents, sterilizes non-disposables, re-assembles them into packs of instruments, towels, gowns and gloves, wraps them in paper and sticks them together with tape, sends them in trains of trucks pulled by electric tractors to the supplies store, whence they are delivered to the user in boxes and trolleys. It is situated in the subterranean regions where so many of our key workers are located. It may have seemed a good idea during the 1950s, but now it looks like a prison where the staff protest at their claustrophobic hole in the ground by a high sickness rate and a high turnover.

Each surgical team probably has two theatres going for each list—one where the consultant does the bigger cases and one where the registrar or senior registrar does some lesser ones. There may be four fairly major cases on one list, which means it will almost certainly over-run: and six or seven very minor operations on the other, which will probably finish on time. The instrument room is shared by the two scrub nurses. A degree of camaraderie and of chit-chat and banter between, and even during, operations is to be expected when people work together over a long period of time. The traditional hierarchy owes more to the market place than it does to science. It remains true that patients from the highest and wealthiest strata of society expect their family doctor to make sure that their private operation is performed by a surgeon of national or international repute. They do not expect to know the name of the anaesthetist, but trust the surgeon to choose someone first class to anaesthetize for him. The same applies in NHS and university circles—the identity of the cardiac or transplant surgeon may be a household name, but who has heard of the anaesthetist? No GP ever says 'I'd like you to be anaesthetized by Dr X, and I'm sure he'll choose a perfectly competent surgeon to do the cutting'. Playing second fiddle is becoming something of a festering sore to the anaesthesiologists, who do, after all, see to the overall life support of the patient and whose skills are delivering increasingly exciting advances in the fields of intensive care and the relief of intractable pain.

Furthermore, each anaesthetist probably spends six or seven sessions a week in theatre, plus emergencies, whereas each surgeon will only have two to four regular theatre lists and will spend the rest of his time in the out-patients' clinic or doing his ward rounds, so the overall management of the theatre suite is increasingly falling to the nursing hierarchy and the anaesthetists. The type of anaesthesia given varies from specialty to specialty, so each consultant will work with perhaps three or four surgeons within the same broad range of specialties. Patients are becoming older and frailer, so spinal and epidural anaesthesia are being used increasingly. This is suitable for operations on the lower extremities, the pelvis and the legs, and involves an injection of local anaesthetic into the fluid surrounding the spinal cord or around the sensory nerves as they emerge from the spinal canal. The former is quick and easy but liable to cause problems if the local anaesthetic is allowed to reach the higher levels of the cord or brain-stem, the latter is difficult technically. Both leave the patient conscious and liable to become bored and uncomfortable if the surgical procedure is a protracted one. Both have many advantages if the lungs or heart are not functioning very well. They can be used in conjunction with a sedative or a light general anaesthetic (GA) which may combine the best of both worlds. Some procedures are carried out entirely under local anaesthesia. In most centres, most operations are still performed using general anaesthesia administered, after the initial 'knock-out' i.v. injection, via the airways. There is, again, a deal of variation between consultants, and many simply insert an artificial airway between the tongue and the palate and squeeze away on a bag connecting the gas bottles to a mask held over the nose and jaw. Others prefer to slip a tube over the back of the tongue and down through the larynx and trachea. For abdominal and thoracic surgery, muscular relaxation is essential, so the patient is paralysed pharmacologically and is therefore unable to breathe. This makes it essential to intubate the patient who will clearly require mechanical ventilation until the effects of the muscle relaxant wear off. One group of patients who are deliberately over-ventilated are the neurosurgical cases in whom it is essential to eliminate as much carbon dioxide as possible from the blood to reduce any brain swelling. For all these more complex procedures, the anaesthetist has what the Americans call the 'vital signs' constantly monitored, so that if the pulse, blood pressure, or carbon dioxide level varies outside predetermined limits, an alarm signal is given and appropriate action is taken. Each consultant anaesthetist at the RI has about seven theatre sessions a week working with three or four different surgical teams. The other sessions are mainly taken up by on-call work, since they frequently have to come in at night. There might be, on average, two emergency operations at night, plus another in maternity and another in the neurosurgery department: the latter is likely to last for four or five hours.

In some respects, the house surgeon is the lowest form of life in the green jungle of the operating theatres, mainly because he is the most transitory.

Hugh, 25, is a senior house officer currently spending six months in my department: his previous job was that of pre-registration house surgeon on a general firm at the RI.

I worked for two consultants, both general surgeons but one of them liked to do some vascular work. I was on take about twice a week and every third weekend and we used to have three or four admissions a night and perhaps one of them would need to go straight to theatre because of a perforated ulcer or a strangulated hernia, or a suspected acute appendix. The registrar or SR would be on with me and he would decide to go ahead and he would do the operation unless it was something really enormous like a bleeding aneurysm when he would call the chief. My job was to contact the theatre staff and call the anaesthetist—again the registrar, who in turn called his consultant if he felt he needed to. The rest of the time I had to clerk the patients on the ward and arrange any investigations and deal with any post-operative complications. And I had to arrange the lists, four of them a week, which meant notifying the theatre staff and making sure that the blood was ordered in advance: two or four units (500 ml in each) for a gastrectomy, one or two for a gall bladder, four for a bowel resection, two for a mastectomy, two for a thyroid, ten or twelve for an aneurysm. And I had to arrange the list so that it was about the right length, three to four medium-length cases, and that they were in the right order—major cases before minor ones, clean cases before dirty ones, young patients before the old, and private before anything. I used to scrub but I only did a couple of cases myself, appendicectomies, which I was talked through by the registrar. I enjoyed it. In fact, I wanted to go on with surgery, but I was no good at it because I can only see at all well with one eye so I have not got three dimensional vision. I used to miss the loose ends of the chief's knots with the scissors, and one day I accidentally cut the knot he had just tied, and afterwards he took me on one side and told me surgery was not for me. He was quite kind about it, really.

The specialized surgeons generally employ junior staff who are on course for a surgical career themselves. Urology is much more than old men with prostates: it is cancer of the kidney and bladder, it is children with malformation of the bladder and ureters, it is pain and obstruction and possible kidney damage caused by stones. Eye and ENT work is mainly carried out under an operating microscope (cost £30K) with a TV screen displaying the proceedings to the assembled company. The eye theatre is in use four and a half days a week and the bread and butter of ophthalmology is cataract treatment, which accounts for an eighth of our out-patient appointments and half the department's operations. Most of the patients are over 70, and the condition is essentially a degenerative one in which the lens becomes progressively opacified and eventually requires removal either under general or local anaesthesia. The duration of stay is usually under a week, and our eye specialists are increasingly implanting artificial lenses to correct the vision instead of supplying the traditional pebble glasses which lead to so much distortion.

A wide range of other eye surgery is carried out, including 100–150 corneal transplants a year. The tough protective coat of the front of the eye can lose its transparency when damaged as a result of inborne defects which become apparent in adult life, or following injuries, virus infections, or unsuccessful cataract surgery. Grafting a cornea from a donor is successful in 85–90 per cent of cases, and unlike other organs, the eye need not be removed until six or even eight hours after death so the ethical issues which beleaguer the criteria of brain death do not arise. The conventional donor, e.g. a young victim of a road traffic accident, is preferred but the supply is insufficient and eyes from people of 60 or even 70 or more are sometimes used. The technique has been available for some decades and it is estimated that quite a number of 100-year-old corneas are still in use, and that one or two will soon reach the age of 120.

Orthopaedics is a large and busy part of the surgical empire and trauma accounts for about half the cases. During a weekend at the RI perhaps 10 patients will need to go to theatre, of whom half will be old ladies (rarely men) who have fallen and sustained fractures of the upper end (neck) of the femur. This particular problem is reaching epidemic proportions and is growing out of proportion to the ageing of the population. By the age of 85, almost 15 per cent of women will have fractured their femoral necks. Old people are liable to fall and their bones are brittle. They are also liable to post-operative complications and the mortality is quite significant (about 15 per cent) and hospital stay is prolonged (about three weeks on average) while the physiotherapists rehabilitate them and arrangements are made for discharge. The fracture is fixed by inserting a nail through the bone, or by replacing the head of the femur by a metal substitute, and every effort is made to get the patient walking on it the following day. The operation is likely to take about two hours, so the workload is considerable. There are also the traffic accident victims and those who have broken bones during various leisure pursuits who may need an operation or who may be encased in plaster and who need observation for a day or two to make sure the limb stays healthy. The other half of the caseload is called 'cold' or 'elective' surgery and includes total hip replacement (THR) which has offered relief from pain to so many arthritic patients over the past 20 years. Not all orthopaedic surgery is of the hammer and chisel variety and not all orthopaedic surgeons rose to riches through valour on the rugger field: restoring function to injured hands and replacing ligaments in the knee with artificial ones calls for delicacy as great as any branch of surgery. However, enough blood gets splashed about during most orthopaedic lists for the surgeons to catch the occasional drop in the eye, and the 'orthopods', the urologists and the neurosurgeons are considering wearing protective goggles because you never know which of your patients is a carrier of the AIDS virus. Another possible source of infection is an accidental prick from a needle which has been used to administer a local anaesthetic (a common enough occurrence), but it has to be said that in the present state of knowledge the risk to health service personnel appears to be extraordinarily small.

The rising tide of trauma cases requiring operations is outstripping the general increase in the demand for surgery, which is itself a great reflection not so much of a decline in health of an ageing population but of the expanding possibilities that surgery has to offer. In 1975 the total number of cases operated on in all theatres was 13 600 and this rose by 40 per cent to 19 200 in 1985, in spite of the development of a nearby hospital which was expected to deflect some of the work. Trauma cases operated on during a comparable period rose by over 75 per cent from 710 to 1260. One of the success stories from the point of view of health care delivery over the past decade has been the growth of day surgery. With the wisdom of hindsight, we thought rather too small when we constructed a day surgery suite with just one theatre. Its use has grown from 550 cases in 1975 to over 2800 in 1985. Patients arrive fasting but with no other preparation, and are anaesthetized, operated on, come round in the recovery room, and return home with their spouse or parent and a set of stitches and a neat bundle of bandage. Lumps, bumps, cysts, varicose veins, amputations of a finger or a toe, cystoscopy, termination of pregnancy, dilatation and curettage of the womb, male sterilization, some laparoscopic female sterilizations (see Chapter 9), and a few hernia repairs are among the operations that can be conveniently carried out on a day basis. In general, this arrangement suits the patients and suits the hospital management. It also suits the surgeons because they can undertake more surgery and leave the major part of the post-operative care to the general practitioner and the community nurse. Surgeons like operating, they have been trained to operate, and operating is what they do best.

7

Sophistication:
Coronary care, intensive care

Being the on-call medical registrar is a fairly high-stress occupation for 24 or 48 hours. There is the stress of never being quite certain what bizarre, unfamiliar, life-threatening condition the local population is going to present you with next, and whether you are going to be able to handle it. The stress of being called to one emergency while in the middle of handling another, and of necessity practising a kind of triage—under pressure you leave the irretrievable, you ignore those who are going to get better anyway, and you focus your efforts on those in whom prompt treatment will critically affect the outcome. There is the stress of having no beds, and still the sick keep coming— so you have to 'borrow' a bed from a resentful surgical firm. There is the stress of cajoling some co-operation out of your colleagues: you may need surgical advice, or the help of the X-ray department or the laboratories, or some extra nursing. The stress of arguing the toss with very senior, very grumpy GPs who do not understand the bed shortage and imply that it is all your fault anyway. Quite simply, the stress of too much work, too much responsibility, too little sleep. The stress of the little black radio-paging device (the bleep or bleeper) which emits its imperious, high-pitched whine as soon as your head is cushioned on the pillow summoning you to ward or phone. However, one of the most stressful events of all is the strident note of the other bleep which you carry around for the day. The second bleep is red, and is reserved for one class of call only, the 'crash call' which indicates a cardiac arrest. A cardiac arrest is the sudden cessation of the circulation of the blood because the heart, through one electrical mechanism or another, and generally due to coronary artery disease, has ceased to beat effectively. It is a different event to a patient dying because of untreatable disease: it is abrupt, it happens to people who are otherwise perfectly sound, and it is potentially salvageable. In the memorable words of one of the pioneers of cardiopulmonary resuscitation (CPR), it happens to 'hearts that are too good to die'.

When a cardiac arrest occurs, it is occasionally a junior doctor but more often a nurse who is on the spot to make the diagnosis (simple— if the patient collapses abruptly, if the main arterial pulse cannot be detected, you have an 'arrest situation'). She commences CPR and shouts to a colleague to run to the 'phone. A fundamental rule in hospitals is that you never run, it upsets the other patients and the visitors. Never in medicine, means hardly ever, so, even in an emergency as hot as this, people usually stride rapidly and only rarely break into a surreptitious run. The person detailed dials 111, the switchboard operator answers instantaneously, is informed simply the location of the arrest, and issues a crash call which triggers the bleeps carried by the essential staff members and informs them ceaselessly where they are needed. The medical registrar on call, the medical house officer on call, a duty anaesthetic registrar, and a specially trained nurse are the key people, and they drop whatever they are doing and proceed at something between a fast lope and a fast jog to the scene of the emergency. The other key person is the duty porter, and he has to collect the 'crash cart' before he can make his way to the ward or A&E department or wherever, again at a frantic yet studiously unhurried pace. The team assemble and take over from the infinitely relieved ward staff who have meanwhile been heroically applying external cardiac massage and mouth-to-mouth respiration to the insensible recumbent figure of the unfortunate victim who has usually been placed upon the floor. The crash trolley contains the essential tools of the trade: cardiac monitor, DC electrical defibrillator, airways, ventilating bags, and an array of drugs and fluids for intravenous administration. The monitor reveals the nature of the electrical disturbance. The defibrillator delivers an electric shock which will depolarize the heart. Following this the heart, having an astonishing propensity to beat rhythmically and indefinitely, will, it is hoped, resume the habitual even tenor of its ways, and then, in the approximately 50 per cent of cases in whom all has gone according to plan, the patient recovers consciousness. He will then, in all probability, be transferred to the Coronary Care Unit (CCU) in case it happens again. The stress of the whole scene of controlled panic is due to the fact that the attending staff have three minutes in which to restore an effective circulation before irreversible brain damage occurs through lack of oxygen. It is also due to the likely observation of a somewhat chaotic and distressing scene by other patients, relatives, and nurses. Furthermore, the whole sequence of events is a highly probable feature of the day since it occurs, on average, rather more often than once every 24 hours.

The CCU, by contrast, is a haven of tranquillity, partly induced by
the heroin which is the single most important treatment for most MI
(myocardial infarction—heart attack or coronary thrombosis) victims.
It comprises six partitioned-off beds within a mixed cardiac and
general medical ward. The visitor usually encounters nothing more
dramatic than six somnolent figures snoozing on their beds. True,
they are mostly connected up to various bits of gadgetry, but they look
undamaged. The CCU is like flying: 95 per cent boredom, and 5 per
cent panic. Most of the patients have come straight from A&E or
admissions, rather than from other wards. Where possible, all
patients referred in with probable MI are sent via the admissions unit
to CCU, as are the 999 ambulance calls who come to A&E and are
then seen by the medical registrar who makes a provisional diagnosis
of MI.

Myocardial infarction was only identified in 1911 and was not
diagnosed clinically until 1927, but cardiovascular disease is by far
the biggest killer in all Western countries with CHD easily outstripping
strokes within that group. (The Japanese, curiously, suffer more
strokes than heart attacks.) If a sample of 1000 British men aged
between 50 and 59 were kept under observation for five years, 25
would die from CHD, 18 of them outside hospital (mainly at home),
15 before the arrival of medical help, 13 within one hour of the onset of
symptoms, and a further 39 would survive MIs of whom 35 would be
admitted to hospital.

This condition often pursues an uncomplicated course and after the
initial chest pain many sufferers heal up well to form a firm fibrous
scar which interferes very little with the action of the heart or the
activity of the victim. Others suffer complications of which life-
threatening disturbances of heart rhythm are among the commonest
in those hearts whose muscle is not irreparably damaged. These
irregular, inefficient heart rhythms are most likely to occur immediately after the attack and the incidence declines thereafter. The
greatest toll therefore is during the period immediately following the
attack, and major campaigns have been launched in the United States
and more recently in the United Kingdom to educate the public in the
techniques of CPR. Unfortunately, these can be counterproductive
unless equal care is taken to ensure that the diagnosis of cardiac arrest
is made with equal proficiency. If no member of the public can sustain
the circulation until effective cardiac activity is restored, the task falls
to the ambulance crew, and in some localities they can actually
diagnose and treat the underlying electrical fault (see Chapter 4). If it

is a question of life support, as it certainly is in most centres including our own, the next best option is rapid admission to the CCU. At the RI we do not have a rush-in facility because we feel that the patient is best served by being seen by the duty registrar in A&E or admissions. Anyone suspected of an MI has an electrocardiogram (ECG) carried out at once and has a cardiac monitor connected up. They are then under constant surveillance from the time of arrival and if the diagnosis is seriously entertained, probably reach CCU about two hours after seeking assistance. Once installed on CCU, all patients are on cardiac monitors which give a constant display of the ECG, and which are linked to a visual display unit (VDU) in the nursing station so that every patient's rate and rhythm is under constant observation. They also have a continuous digital read-out of the rate and alarms are triggered off if it varies above or below pre-determined limits, so immediate action can be taken. This is likely to consist of the application of the two electrode paddles to the chest by one of the nurses whose colleague operates the switch to deliver a shock of 300 joules. There are two specially trained nurses permanently on duty: the doctors may not be nearly so instantaneously available, so the nurses have to be able to act on their own initiative. The first priority is restoring circulation; the next, ventilation: everything else can wait, although not for long. The doctors, when they arrive, put up i.v. lines and run in bicarbonate to counteract the rapid build-up of acid caused by oxygen starvation. They may need to inject drugs which act on the heart in order to speed it up or slow it down. They may need to insert a temporary pacemaker if the rate is too slow, or to ventilate the lungs mechanically, if profound unconsciousness is prolonged.

There were 560 admissions to CCU last year but already 315 in the first six months of this year which must reflect a change in usage rather than a true rise in the incidence of MI. For instance, some cases of self-poisoning with antidepressant drugs cause life-threatening disturbances of the heart beat. There are also patients who are subsequently found to have some totally different disorder more suitably looked after elsewhere. The unit is generally full, so beds are found for newcomers by moving one of the existing occupants to a general medical ward. The usual duration of stay is 36 or 48 hours. An educated guess would be that 50 deaths occur on CCU during a year, and perhaps 50 or 100 patients are salvaged from what would otherwise have been a fatal event. The risk of these electrical disturbances which stop the pumping action of the heart declines steadily after the initial MI, but occasionally patients do arrest after their return to the general ward, and if the outcome of the crash call is successful, they will usually go back to the CCU and start again, rather like a lethal game of snakes and ladders.

In spite of the usual narcotic torpor of the place, CCU is medical tiger country. The surgeons and anaesthetists also have their tiger country, but it is usually a scene of appropriately frenetic activity. This is the intensive therapy (or treatment, or care) unit (ITU) which is a 12-bedded annex to one of the surgical wards on the same level as the operating suite. There is some overlap in function, but CCU is more to maintain the action of the heart, ITU, that of the lungs. Surgeons are seldom seen on CCU: physicians are often encountered on ITU, although they are not entirely at home there—it is really the domain of the anaesthetists, with their tubes down peoples' windpipes and their electrical machines which link to these tubes and blow the lungs up and down. Some of the more massive post-operative care is carried out in ITU, after resuscitating a moribund patient whose aorta has ruptured and been repaired, after removing most of the gullet, after massive trauma in some terrible accident, and after certain transplantation procedures. The medical patients would be those with respiratory failure, for example, people with bad chests during an influenza outbreak or profoundly comatose after massively overdosing with sedative drugs, or unable to use the respiratory muscles due to a paralysing disease of the nervous system. Not all the inmates are on ventilators by any means, but many are on drips, transfusions, continuous drug infusion pumps, cardiac monitoring, dialysis, or epidural anaesthesia. It will be appreciated from the nature of the caseload, that much of the work is much 'dirtier' than it is in the CCU in that infection is much commoner and may be overwhelming in patients in such a parlous state, and it is often caused by particularly virulent strains of bacteria. Infection seems to occur in outbreaks, especially when the unit is crowded because space is short in view of all the equipment surrounding each bed. After all, the hands of doctors, nurses, and others who handle patients are probably the most important vehicles of cross-infection.

The condition of some of the patients comes as a surprise to the visitor because a few of them are sitting feeding themselves, perhaps breathing through tracheostomies (holes directly through the neck into the windpipe). These people are probably being 'weaned off' their ventilators, since once a function such as respiration has been taken over by mechanical means, it takes a little time before the centres of the brain-stem can resume the activity without a little fine-tuning.

Although often under great pressure, ITU enjoys something of a 'boom–slump' economy with periods of relative respite. The nursing level is high, with a one-to-one ratio, and the staff quickly find that relief turns to boredom when the unit becomes quiet.

In 1986 ITU accepted 300 patients with an average duration of stay, before returning to the general wards, of six days. Of these, 50 died on the ITU, and 200 were ventilated. Deaths are commonly due to infection, inability to maintain nutrition, acute renal failure, and brain damage. The medical staff consist of three consultant anaesthetists who take it in turn to be nominally in charge, two medical registrars and a senior registrar, and an anaesthetic registrar and senior registrar who alternate and sleep in when on duty. A casual visit revealed the following patients: man, 42, lung damage due to smoke from burning car; female, 31, toxic shock; man, 30, gunshot wound to chest and liver; two patients following surgery to heart and aorta; man, traffic accident, fractured ribs and punctured lungs on both sides (and thus likely to need assisted respiration); woman, 25, overdose; woman, 52, polyneuritis with ascending paralysis.

We started this chapter by talking about stress, and perhaps it is reasonable to end it on the same note. The nurses on the ITU undergo a great deal of stress, especially when there is a run of deaths, and the sister in charge identifies psychological counselling as one of the unmet needs of her staff. Much the same applies to CCU, where there is a similar potential for maintaining life by the skilled handling of technology until nature or medical intervention succeeds or fails in its endeavour to repel the threat. But what about the patients? Are they mercifully too clouded by drugs and disease to appreciate how precarious their predicament and how total their dependence? One simple but striking enquiry showed that during the day noise level in one busy London ITU was equivalent to that of heavy street traffic, with an aggravatingly loud noise occurring every two minutes or so. It has also been shown that a number of patients subsequently recall vivid hallucinations, no doubt due to a mixture of chemical assaults on the brain by medication and disordered metabolism and bacterial action. Sleep deprivation is a contributory factor, and it is perhaps surprising that not a great deal of attention is paid in the literature to the simple question of how aware are patients in CCU and ITU that they are poised on the brink of dissolution, and how terrified are they of slipping over that brink into the abyss beyond? Such questions are difficult to address until after the event; and after the event, some merciful natural mechanism swiftly obliterates such morbid preoccupations from our minds. For the majority who survive desperate illnesses thanks to CCUs and ITUs, their major subsequent anxieties revert to the perennial demands of the Inland Revenue, the Hire Purchase Company, the Building Society, and the City or County Treasurer.

8

The glittering heights: Neurosurgery, transplant, and cardiac surgery

To use the current jargon, some kinds of medicine are sexy and some are not. Into the latter category fall community medicine, psychiatry, geriatrics, dermatology, and probably anaesthetics. It is just as well that today's youngsters are too mature to be lured into the profession by such trivial considerations, since we need far more of these hewers of wood and drawers of water than we do of the whizz-kids with the glamorous Dr Kildare image. It is also an exceedingly arduous route to the glittering heights of the superstar specialties for the ascent is so competitive that total commitment is the essential requisite. The three specialties that spring to mind as enjoying the highest status in the public consciousness are neurosurgery, transplant surgery, and cardiac surgery. All three are regional specialties, and are therefore located at the RI, where the first two have their own blocks off the main ground floor corridor.

Neurosciences, to give its official title, is located next to radiology (see Chapter 11) because of the extensive demands it makes on that department and in particular on head scanning. On the ground floor is the head injury ward of 14 beds including a small four-bedded neuro-intensive therapy unit (ITU). These head injury patients will be the bad ones, from all over the region, and not the minor ones from the city admitted for observation after falling off a step-ladder and getting knocked out. It is therefore a ward with a high level of tragedy since the occupants are usually young and were entirely healthy until a passing container truck wreaked random havoc with their lives. Some of those being ventilated in the ITU will either fail to recover consciousness, or will do so only to be found to have sustained brain damage. The former patients eventually die and become a source of organs for the transplant team. The latter suffer from permanent physical, mental, or personality defects and become a source of almost equal sorrow to their families or, if requiring too much care to go home, worry to the hospital staff as there is no provision for their longer-term care.

Upstairs is a 24-bed ward including four more ITU beds mainly for post-operative care, and above that, two more 24-bed wards, one containing a small children's unit of six cots and the other devoted mainly to medical neurology. Finally, the top floor houses two operating theatres where the four consultants share nine lists a week between them.

Much of the workload is traumatic and arrives during unsocial hours following antisocial behaviour. Operations to lift depressed skull fractures or to evacuate great clots of blood or abscesses that are compressing vital brain tissue often last for several hours. Some are relatively quick and easy, and collections of blood lying between brain and skull can be drained through simple burr-holes. Most neuro-surgical procedures, whether 'hot' or 'cold' (i.e. urgent or elective), are designed to relieve pressure on the brain or the spinal cord, whether by a benign but slowly enlarging tumour or by a disc protruding from between two of the neck vertebrae. Sometimes the pressure comes from within and the ventricles deep in the cerebral hemispheres which contain the clear cerebrospinal fluid start expand-ing and a shunt has to be inserted to conduct the fluid away. Other operations concern the cerebral arteries, for example, when a defect in one of them bursts to release a torrent of blood which must be stemmed, or when the blood supply is threatened and needs to be augmented. A patient of mine admitted with a heart attack was discovered by an assiduous house physician to be unable to see outside of the midline from either eye, totally unknown to the gentleman concerned who had been cycling around the city oblivious to overtaking juggernauts. X-rays confirmed a pituitary tumor (at the base of the brain) pressing on the optic nerves and this was in due course successfully removed by a neurosurgeon. The skull is a rigid box, and pressure building up within it must be relieved to prevent damage to fragile but vital brain tissue, and this simple fact is the key to neurosurgery.

Transplant surgery is one of the rapidly advancing fields of medical endeavour, and has achieved a high degree of success for patients with kidneys that have stopped working (see Chapter 5), for whom it is the most cost-effective form of treatment. Forty recipients attend each weekly follow-up clinic, and most of them are extraordinarily good advertisements for the operation and lead unrestricted lives. When a kidney does become available, it arrives in a cardboard box packed in crushed ice and it then takes five or seven hours of testing in the tissue-typing laboratory to make sure of its acceptibility. Should the tests be unfavourable, it starts off on its travels again to the next centre and the average kidney undergoes one to two (actually 1½) of these journeys. The unwritten rules are that when you have a donor, you take one of the kidneys for local use and the other one is offered nation-wide.

We do 70 or more transplants a year but would do more if a larger proportion of the perfectly good kidneys, which are buried or cremated with their tragically deceased owners was made available. In March 1986, there were 3303 patients waiting for kidney transplantation in the United Kingdom and the Republic of Ireland compared with 249 for hearts and 75 for livers. The national requirement is probably about 2,500 annually and, in fact, 1600 were carried out in 1986. We can boast that in the United Kingdom there are an estimated 5773 living recipients of functioning kidneys, which is more than any other European country.

One or two pancreas plus kidney transplants for diabetic patients have been carried out at the RI, but there are technical difficulties still to be overcome. The guidelines concerning organ donation at the RI indicate that anyone dying without sepsis, malignant disease, kidney disease, high blood pressure or diabetes qualifies for consideration although, in practice, organs from people over 70 are not regarded as suitable. Head injury deaths afford the richest source of organs and it will be necessary to request permission from the coroner, and also the next of kin unless the deceased person is carrying a kidney donor card and has thus given his own permission in advance. Liver transplantation is a very much more formidable undertaking than kidney grafting and the demand is not nearly so great, although we are hoping to start our own programme shortly. It is very worthwhile in a few highly selected cases in whom it is not only immediately life saving but sometimes brings many years of extra life. At the time of writing the longest survivor underwent the operation over 11 years ago, and about 60 per cent of adults and 70 per cent of children are alive at one year although a third of treated children need a second graft. The pioneer in this field is the Professor of Surgery at one of our ancient universities and he runs what is called a supraregional service (approximately 65 transplants annually) which effectively means that he does nearly all the liver transplants for the United Kingdom as well as a significant number for other European countries. I was fortunate enough to meet one of the key members of his staff the day after a rather hectic 24 hours of activity by the team.

Carol: Regional Transplant Co-ordinator

I was a nurse and became involved in this work after spending three years with the renal unit. My job is a very varied one and often quite distressing because I am usually the person who has to approach the relatives to ask them if they would be willing to allow us to use the organs and I have to do this pretty well immediately after death. You really have to believe in what you are doing, to do that. Most of the donors have come from either the ITU or neurosurgery, and they usually let me know in advance when they have a potential donor on the ward.

We practically always have somebody waiting for a liver transplant and the operation can go ahead as soon as a liver becomes available via the UK Transplant Service in Bristol. Our patients have to spend a few days in hospital undergoing all the preliminary work-up, but after that we keep them out of hospital as much as possible and I try to get the family accommodated locally in a bed-and-breakfast establishment because it may be the last time they will have, to spend together as a family. Unfortunately, they have to pay for this themselves, we do not have the funds to help them. Sometimes the patient is in hospital and is so sick that the transplant is required urgently and then we contact various national transplant services to seek a suitable liver. In France, for instance, they have this high degree of discipline whereby when the organs become available, even if they have a recipient waiting locally, they will contact the national service before going ahead just in case there is someone in more desperate need waiting elsewhere, even in a different country, and then that patient will take priority.

When a liver does become available we have a maximum of eight hours for which it can be preserved before it is grafted into place but if it can be done sooner, so much the better. [A kidney can be kept viable for 24 hours, but a heart must be removed and implanted within three hours]. Yesterday, for instance, we had this very ill girl in hospital in severe liver failure and she was not going to live another 24 hours without a transplant. She was already a recipient a few months ago and she had thrombosed her hepatic artery so the liver was necrotic [dead]. At about 11 in the morning I heard that a donor had become available in France. We said thank you very much, could we please remove the liver ourselves because we prefer it that way, and I assembled the team. This time it was four people, the professor's assistant, who has been fully trained-up for transplantation work, a junior surgeon, a scrub nurse, and the organ technician. We organized a small jet from the local airport, but of course when they came back they had to land at an international airport to clear customs. They bring it back in an ice-box, you know? just like the ones you use for a picnic, and it is immersed in ice and saline. The police fetched them from the airport, we find they are quite extraordinarily helpful.

Meanwhile, the professor was flying back from a conference in Helsinki, so I had to contact the conference, the airline, and Heathrow to get the message through that when he landed he was to come straight to theatre and we went ahead and had the girl in there and being worked on before the liver had actually landed. She went in at about 10.30 in the evening, and I believe that it was a 10 hour operation—they usually take nearer six.

We always make sure that 30 units of blood are available, and often use 10. I believe the record is 400 and is held by an American team. Until his assistant arrived a couple of years ago, the professor had to do it all himself, both the organ removal and the grafting procedures. I do not think he could possibly do that now because we are doing well over 60 a year.. Most of the livers come from this country, of course, and then it is much simpler because we can use helicopters which can get much nearer to the donor's hospital as well as being able to land right in the grounds here.

Most of the donors are going to give multiple organs—liver, kidneys, possibly heart and pancreas, corneas—and we depend very much on the attitudes of the medical staff who looked after them in life as well as those of the families. I think opinion is swinging in our favour, although I recognize that some people even here feel very threatened by us. I never go onto one of the wards here unless I'm invited, never . . .

To give an idea of the scale of transplant surgery in the United Kingdom, during the first six months of 1986, 797 kidney transplants were performed, 103 hearts (or heart and lungs), and 56 livers.

My brother had the misfortune to be a patient in the RI when the usual clamour in the ward was eclipsed by the sound of a helicopter landing outside. A figure was seen scurrying below the still rotating blades carrying a small case in either hand. 'Wonderful' remarked the ward domestic, 'Here comes the professor with a couple of kidneys from a transplant operation on a North Sea oil rig'. The truth was much less exciting—it was Father Christmas arriving to commence duty at one of our major department stores.

Heart surgery is difficult to separate from the medical specialty of cardiology, and even harder to separate from the surgical specialty of thoracic (mainly lung) surgery since it tends to be lumped together under the all-embracing term 'cardiothoracic surgery'. What happens is that the cardiologists have a ward in which, amongst other things, they 'work-up' patients to present for cardiac surgery, and the chest physicians have a ward in which, amongst other things, they 'work-up' patients to present for lung surgery. They share a specialized X-ray facility and the surgeons share a theatre, an ITU, and a ward. The chest physicians provide a semi-Regional service and investigate all those who might be possible candidates for excision of a lung or a lobe of a lung, almost invariably because of cancer. Only a minority of sufferers from this complaint are suitable for an attempt at surgical cure. This may be because the position of the tumour is unfavourable or the nature of it is too malignant, or it has already spread elsewhere, or the general condition of the patient, or that of the remaining lung tissue (since the vast majority have been smokers) will not sustain life following lung resection. Nevertheless, for this fortunate minority the procedure is not too daunting and the results are favourable with 50–80 per cent of the cases treated surviving four years. 100–150 of these operations are performed annually.

Cardiology has all the features of a high-prestige specialty. It is extremely competitive, it is very easy to fall off the ladder, and consultants are above the average age at appointment. The technology is highly skilled and rapidly advancing, there is a body of hard knowledge poorly understood by the rest of the profession and the diseases they deal with are often matters of life or death. In addition, there is a considerable amount of private practice. Cardiologists provide a truly regional service and roam the far-flung outposts of the empire doing clinics and seeing those unfortunate captives of the other DGHs 50 miles or more away that are defeating the skills of their own consultants or have been assessed by them as requiring some form of intervention. Sometimes they simply give advice to the local team, some of these patients they will transfer to the RI, and other patients are transferred into cardiology at the RI urgently after a telephone discussion between referring hospital and cardiology registrar. Usually, the cardiac ward is a 'cold' ward; although often seriously ill, few of the patients are red hot emergencies, and, as explained elsewhere, the majority of cardiac emergencies such as coronaries and acute heart failure come in under the on-take physician or geriatrician.

Admissions to cardiology number about 1500 a year. Two or three hundred are related to the pacemaker service and we fit 150 a year. These admissions are usually in and out in five days: one day to have it inserted (under general anaesthetic and X-ray control) and four days to make sure it works well and the wound heals over. Of the rest, some are abnormalities of heart rhythm which have proved resistant to the conventional drug treatment administered by the general physicians. A few are infections of the heart valves requiring prolonged and often massive antibiotic regimes if irreparable damage to the valves is to be avoided. A fair number are patients with damaged valves who need assessment for open-heart (valve replacement) surgery. The majority are victims of coronary artery disease (coronary heart disease, CHD), mostly suffering from cardiac pain, who undergo coronary arteriography by either cardiologist or radiologist. A fine flexible cannula is fed up the brachial or femoral artery until its tip is opposite the mouth of the coronary arteries and contrast is injected and its course through the coronaries followed by cine-radiography. Approximately 900 coronary arteriograms are performed annually. If an accessible, solitary narrowing can be identified, an attempt may be made to widen it by passing a balloon-tipped catheter into the narrowed segment and inflating it. Otherwise, the patient may be offered coronary artery bypass grafting (CABG).

About 500 cardiology admissions are presented to the surgeons each year, two-thirds of them for CABG, which accounts for over 300 of the 550 annual open-heart operations. All the cardiothoracic surgical patients arrive via the specialist physicians, and not only do the GPs not have direct access to the surgeons but neither do the general physicians. A CABG operation takes two or three hours and valve replacement rather longer, so only about three cases go to theatre daily. There will be about 14 people in the theatre including technicians to man the pump which maintains the circulation while the heart is stopped. The anaesthetists tend to do this type of work for a limited period and then, finding it too demanding, withdraw: the surgeons love it and are quite insatiable. The spare parts used in CABG are segments of vein from the patient's leg or a length of chest-wall artery, those used for valve replacement are artificial. Most of the valves are aortic, and these days they have generally become diseased and obstruct the outflow of blood simply through wear and tear, so the subjects are often quite elderly.

It all sounds very glamorous but it has actually become quite routine. After surgery, the patient generally spends 48 hours being monitored in the six-bed cardiothoracic intensive therapy unit and then a few days in the surgical ward. The surgery is elective rather than urgent, the complication rate of CABG is only 25 per cent and the mortality rate an amazing 1 per cent. In the United States it has become a more common operation than appendicectomy (appendectomy, US usage) and one man in 14 has undergone the procedure by the age of 70. The routine nature of modern heart surgery may partly explain why our cardiac surgeons are so keen to join the bandwagon and start our own heart transplant programme. The rest of the consultants are undecided, hoping on the one hand to attract more resources, funds, staff, and prestige to the RI, but fearing on the other than such a development could prove to be a cuckoo in the nest and gobble up an awful lot of what we already have.

9

Farming people:
Obstetrics, paediatrics

Depending on the direction from which the visitor approaches the RI, he will encounter any one of a number of foothills clustered around the main ward block. One of the more imposing of these is a three-storey structure fronted by a portico bearing the legend 'Maternity Wing'. The purpose of this building is to keep the city populated with a steady supply of new inhabitants. Unlike the other departments of the RI, therefore, it is associated with normal, healthy, happy human activity and this is reflected in the pleasant and informal atmosphere and the colourful and attractive furnishings which are more suggestive of an hotel than a hospital. The entrance lobby is carpeted in beige and brightened by potted ferns, and the young lady at the enquiries desk divides the incoming stream of humanity into the visitors who are despatched upstairs to the wards, and the newly expectant mothers who turn right to the antenatal clinic (ANC). Here they will be booked in at about 14 weeks into the pregnancy, and here they will return at regular intervals until they finally come in at the onset of labour. The emphasis today in ante-natal surveillance is on 'shared care'—shared between the hospital and the GP, so every alternate check-up is carried out in his surgery by the woman's own doctor. Apart from being more convenient, this has the advantage of reducing the workload to manageable proportions. Even so, the ANC generally has 60–80 mothers attending each session to be weighed, to have their urine and blood pressure checked, and the baby prodded and listened to. At about 18 weeks the visit will include a 10 minute ultrasound examination, when the expectant mother lies on a couch in a dimly lit room while the radiographer holds a probe coated with cold jelly against her tummy. An image of the baby emerges on the screen, grainy, only black and white, but amazing in its detail. The eyes are clearly seen, the arms waving feebly, the heart beating, even the valves of the heart opening and closing. The sex of the fetus can be determined with a high degree of accuracy, although various complex ethical and medico-legal issues prevent the information from being made readily available. Special care is taken to examine the spine for any defect, and if the radiographer is not happy that all is well, she will arrange a more detailed examination by one of the radiologists.

There are now perhaps 10 or 15 home confinements in the city and its environs a year. They are frowned upon by the medical establishment, and the women who insist that home is the right place to have their babies are regarded as a little eccentric. All other babies are born in the maternity wing, rather more than 10 a day on the average, and the mothers may come from a radius of about 20 miles (32 km). When the time comes to be admitted they generally telephone through to a midwife who asks the frequency of the contractions and, if they are only occurring every 10 minutes or so, may suggest 'phoning back a little later. Some arrive only to be sent home again, but all are examined first of all in an assessment room before being taken into one of the labour rooms. There is a suite specially set aside for GPs who wish to deliver their own patients, but it is seldom used. There are special labour rooms for the 10 per cent or so who are going to require forceps. The normal deliveries are managed by midwives and it is nowadays rare for anyone to take more than 12 hours to give birth. The labour rooms are as uninstitutional as it is reasonable to expect, and are pleasingly appointed. Emergency requirements such as the oxygen supply are concealed behind the locker, and the clinical ceiling light and the large bowls on trolley wheels are the only obtrusive features that reveal the purpose of the place. Until, that is, the monitoring equipment is wired up so that there is a continuous display of the baby's heart rate and the rate and pressure of the uterine contractions. Perhaps 30 per cent of mothers elect to have an epidural anaesthetic, which is about double the proportion nation-wide because we are one of the 50 per cent of units which offer an epidural on demand. In this procedure, the anaesthetist inserts a fine tube into the fatty space outside the spinal cord and its sheath. Local anaesthetic is injected down it from time to time and will infiltrate around the nerves carrying sensation from the pelvic organs to the cord. It generally causes a degree of temporary weakness of the legs, but this is a small price to pay for a painless delivery and it is increasingly preferred to the traditional use of injections of pethidine and whiffs of Entonox. It is especially useful for delivering twins and for breech presentations. When the action happens, those present in the room are mother, baby, usually father, midwife, and pupil midwife. There are between 90 and 100 midwives on the staff, and they are distinguished from other nurses by their red belts. The medical staff are instantly available if an emergency arises: occasionally one of the mothers has a post-partum haemorrhage requiring a transfusion of 10 units or more of blood. Forceps deliveries are handled by a junior doctor, the lower birth canal being numbed by a nerve block or an epidural anaesthetic.

It is often claimed by the natural childbirth lobby that delivery has become excessively medicalized, and that it is increasingly accelerated in order to take place during reasonably social hours. In fact, only 10 or 15 per cent of births are induced, either by rupturing the membranes or by means of a syntocin infusion. Twelve hours is regarded as the maximum period a first-time mother should be allowed to remain in labour. Some 17 per cent of deliveries take place by Caesarian section, generally when there are mechanical difficulties or evidence of danger to the baby as indicated by the monitor. Many of these operations are now performed using an epidural block rather than under a general anaesthetic. Since the first English mother survived the procedure (Jane Foster of Blackrod, Lancashire, in 1793), the proportion of Caesarean sections has been, and still is, rising all the time for two main reasons. One is the increasingly litigious nature of the public and their legal advisers who are responsible for what the Americans, more used to this scene than ourselves, call 'defensive medicine'. The other reason is that it is a self-perpetuating phenomenon, so that once you have had one Caesarean section, future deliveries are almost certain to be by the same route. Our rate is significantly above the national rate of just over 10 per cent, while that in the United States is nearer 20 per cent. The aim must be to do fewer emergency Caesareans, if at the expense of more planned ones, and this is the policy at the RI.

After mother and baby have been made respectable and introduced to each other, and suitably refreshed, they are taken to their respective resting places—the ward and the nursery. Most strong, healthy young women go home after about 48 hours, although complicated cases stay in longer. Premature infants, in particular, are in this category and are transferred to the special care baby unit (SCBU). Twenty metres of wide, pleasantly carpeted, glass-sided corridor separate the delivery suite from the SCBU with its 24 cots, six of which are grouped into a neonatal ITU. This is where the very premature babies weighing for instance 1.5 to 1.7 kg (around 28 to 30 weeks gestation time and representing about 1.5 per cent of births) are placed because they often have serious lung difficulties although they can usually be salvaged. A number of the so-called very low birth weight babies (1000 to 1500 g) survive, and so do about a half of the 'extremely low birth weight' babies who only weigh in at 600 to 700g after some 26 weeks' pregnancy, although up to a half of the smallest survivors will be handicapped in some way. 23 or 24 weeks seems to be the limit since the weight at this stage is half a kilogram or less. The demands made on medical and nursing time in order to resuscitate these diminutive bundles of precarious life are enormous. The average duration of stay of a baby weighing under 1 kg is 100 days, but if the weight is between 1 kg and 1.5 kg it is down to 40 days. Each cot is a tiny laboratory containing a wizened scrap of humanity attached to a bewildering network of lines, and flanked by instrument dials and drip feed regulators. There is a tube into the nose to ventilate the baby, there is a long venous line and an umbilical arterial line for nutrition, and for monitoring purposes. The parameters observed include the blood pressure, the pulse, the temperature, the inspired oxygen concentration, the blood gases—which are all checked by plentiful and ever-vigilant staff around the clock. The babies are wrapped in polythene to reduce water loss through the skin. The SCBU is where, for example, the occasional sets of quadruplets or quintuplets spend their first two months, and make exceedingly heavy demands on the resources available, especially while occupying the ITU. These multiple births result from the triumphs of hormonal treatment for infertility but are in truth a far from desirable outcome as the babies are so tiny and premature. The mother has to face many weeks of intense anxiety and intense publicity and is lucky to emerge with one or two healthy, normal infants at the end of it all. One of the principal immediate dangers is immaturity of the lungs. A longer-term problem is the risk of mental handicap, and one in three of those weighing under 1 lb 12 oz (786g) are severely subnormal.

Needless to say not every child brought into the world at the RI manages to avoid further contact with it. The children's wards are where it is always Christmas because they are always festooned with Chinese lanterns and hanging aeroplanes and exuberant posters and there are colourful figures on the windows and the visitor trips over undersized tractors with undersized drivers. There are three wards; two of them mainly medical, one for children under three and the other for children aged from three to fourteen, and there is a small intensive care unit with just four beds. The surgical ward is for children requiring operations, mainly orthopaedic, ENT, urological, plastic surgery, general, and occasionally eyes. A battle raged, several years ago, whether these children should should go in with the adults of the same specialty but it was felt that this might easily be a most disturbing experience for them and almost nation-wide the paediatricians have now colonized tracts of infant country. The medical children have a wide range of disorders but some of them crop up again and again. Asthma seems to remain as prevalent as ever and the RI has its own club of regulars. Asthmatic children and their parents are rather like diabetics: they get to know more about their own particular brand of the disease than any doctor. It may be hard enough for the family physician to know whether little Patrick is brewing up for a bad attack or not, let alone the locum appearing on the scene for the first time in the middle of the night. Patrick's mother has a shrewd idea though, and Patrick himself knows for sure. Many hospitals therefore have a special arrangement whereby their asthmatic children can take themselves direct to the ward to save the time involved in calling out the GP. We do not have this arrangement, partly because we enjoy a good relationship of mutual trust with the local practices, partly because the paediatricians believe that immediate treatment with nebulized bronchodilator by the GP is good treatment capable of aborting attacks which would otherwise become severe enough to warrant hospital admission.

The other common ailments of childhood include pneumonitis, gastro-enteritis (inserting an i.v. line in a fretting infant can be a nightmare for both parties), convulsions, meningitis, and diabetes. We also tend to collect a tragic little group of childhood cancers from around the region because of our special expertise, including one or two new cases of leukaemia every month. In addition, there is always a handful of curious inherited disorders of body chemistry. There are five consultant paediatricians, six registrars or senior registrars, and six senior house officers, some of whom are training for general practice and some of whom wish to become career paediatricians. The bed numbers in the wards are a little variable: it is the only area in the hospital where it is permissible to put up extra beds in an emergency. This is not because the beds are smaller so much as because quite a significant amount of the care of these small charges is carried out by their parents. The permanent presence of numerous mothers on the wards is one of the features of life that the nurses and doctors rapidly become accustomed to. Although of such comparatively recent construction, the wards were never built with this in mind because it has been a development of the past 20 years or so. The parents therefore live in conditions of considerable inconvenience in little cubicles with the child or in side-rooms if their child is in a four-bed or six-bed bay. For this, and other reasons, we are most anxious to develop a separate building as a purpose-designed children's hospital on the site. (The reason it is no longer acceptable to put up extra beds in the middle of the adult wards when full is that there has been a belated realization that people are looked after by nurses, not beds. To have more patients than there are staff to manage is to do a disservice to the extra patient, the existing patients, and the staff themselves.) In spite of the generally cheery atmosphere, many of the junior doctors rotating through the department find it a stressful experience. The work is hard, the patients do not welcome their attentions, there is always the need to harbour a lurking suspicion that an injured child has been battered, and the deaths are especially hard to adjust to. There are also the infants with neurological abnormalities such as spina bifida and hydrocephalus requiring shunts to relieve the pressure, and these are not always the most rewarding cases to handle.

Before leaving the world of mothers, babies, and children, there are other aspects of the work of the obstetricians which must be mentioned. Unhappily, some 600–700 abortions are performed every year, mostly in the day-case surgical unit. One in six, or maybe one in four, of the city's pregnancies are terminated, and this is performed by suction up to the age of 14 or even 18 weeks. Individual obstetricians take different standpoints on this issue, but all of ours operate a liberal system which virtually offers abortion on demand. At least this avoids the necessity of the mid-trimester termination, an extremely unpopular procedure which either involves a miniature Caesarean with the delivery of a non-viable infant which the surgeon hates doing, or running in an infusion to precipitate labour, which the nursing staff hate doing. Those few mothers who do wish to terminate an advanced pregnancy are usually referred to a private clinic in a nearby town which carries out a considerable amount of this work. The obstetricians also embrace the sister specialty of gynaecology, which concerns itself with diseases of the female reproductive system. This might give the initial impression of being a somewhat restricted field, and indeed there is a considerable amount of fairly bread-and-butter work which forms the basis of what has always been a notably jam-covered specialty. Their operating lists always include several dilatation and curettage (D&Cs), for instance to identify the cause of post-menopausal bleeding. Hysterectomy comes second equal with termination after D&C, and next would probably be laparoscopic sterilization which involves tubal ligation via an instrument inserted through the abdominal wall just below the umbilicus. This can be done in the day-care surgical unit, and the laparoscope is also used to inspect the ovaries and other organs to investigate infertility or to exclude a tumour or other pathology.

The gynaecologists run the colposcopy service for women whose cervical smear has shown suspicious cells which might be, or might become, malignant. The neck of the womb is inspected by means of a binocular microscope which is directed down the speculum, and samples (biopsies) are taken from abnormal looking areas. If this confirms that malignant change is occurring, a subsequent visit is arranged so that the offending areas can be treated with a laser. This is an important and successful development. The death rate from cancer of the cervix of the uterus has remained constant, while the incidence of premalignant change has increased dramatically, due, it is thought, to the increasingly promiscuous habits of the population. The territory of one specialty invariably overlaps with that of several others, and women with serious pelvic disease are treated by cancer specialists, while those with ruptured ovarian cysts are sometimes operated on by the general surgeons. Vaginal discharges are often the rightful concern of the venereologist, and incontinence of urine may be treated by the urologist. The female pelvis is a crowded area, and some of its problems were vividly described by the senior gynaecologist at my own teaching hospital: 'The trouble with the female anatomy', he declared many years before sexism became an ugly word, 'is that the ignition is situated too near to the exhaust'. The area is also crowded by the number of specialists eager to explore it, particularly perhaps in the private sector. 'Sexual intercourse', a recently retired gynaecologist informed his senior registrar, 'is 30 per cent pleasure and 70 per cent work'. The senior registrar looked puzzled. 'I don't think that can be right', he ventured rather diffidently, 'otherwise I'd be doing all yours for you'.

10

Low tech:
Psychiatry

We view it as something of a disgrace that psychiatric wards at the RI are still, at the time of writing, no more than a gleam in the eye of the professor of psychiatry, and a series of files going back over at least 15 years. Meanwhile, from his office in university country on the RI complex, the professor's journey to his wards takes him southwards until he reaches the motorway, then northwards to bypass the city and finally southwards once again until he enters the outskirts. There, situated in some 50 acres of pleasing lawns and shrubberies, stands as forbidding a pile of Victorian masonry as can be found outside the works of Bram Stoker and Edgar Allen Poe. This is our psychiatric hospital, formerly mental hospital, formerly lunatic asylum, and although a succession of secretaries of state has declared an intention to close down these institutions, the economic climate never quite permits it to be done. There are, it is true, a couple of ward blocks of comparatively recent construction, but they are in some ways more depressing than the main building, having been built to a low specification and systematically neglected ever since so that the woodwork has been left unvarnished and has rotted, there are windows missing, there are holes in the plaster and the roof leaks.

The victims of mental illness have still to achieve acceptance, let alone the sympathy and generosity lavished by the public on the physically sick. The specialty, similarly, is not held in very high esteem in the medical profession which generally feels more comfortable with abnormalities you can measure, and which regards the science of psychiatry as distinctly soft. Add to that a chronically deficient staff working in archaic facilities the wrong side of town and the result is a perfect recipe for low morale, poor standards of care, and recurrent scandals in the local press. It is to the eternal credit of the nurses and doctors who work there that none of this happens and the hospital enjoys a very high reputation in the field of psychiatric care, if a somewhat ambivalent one amongst the local population. They have to be the unsung heroines (and heroes) of the hospital service.

The psychiatric hospital has far too large a catchment area and serves about 500 000 souls because neighbouring districts have never seen fit to provide sufficient resources of their own. This means that there are insufficient beds and all it can provide is an emergency service with scarcely any elective, or waiting list, admissions coming from the clinics. General practitioners find it very hard to admit their patients because there are so few empty beds—the occupancy rate is about 96 per cent. When patients have to be admitted compulsorily (a very small minority—perhaps 20 per cent) it is sometimes necessary to put up extra beds to accommodate them. There are insufficient staff for the number of beds, and it is seldom possible to have a patient 'specialled' by one nurse assigned to supervise him alone, for instance because of a serious threat of suicide. A special nurse will probably have to deal with several high-risk patients at once.

The concept of a hospital bed does not really apply to a psychiatric hospital. In a general hospital, the bed is often the key location because patients may spend some days in bed and are likely to have things done to them in bed, although even then, the concept is a faulty one. Patients are looked after by nurses, not by beds, so it is the number of nurses that determines the number of patients, not the quantity of bedsteads and mattresses. In a psychiatric hospital, none of the patients are in bed. Each ward has a couple of dormitories and perhaps a single cubicle or two. The dormitories are like those of a boy's preparatory school with pathetically little personal terrain and no privacy, and when one visits there is the same unnatural neatness with each bed carefully made and covered with a counterpane. Where are all the patients? Many of them will be in evidence in other areas of the ward, sitting around in groups in one of the day-rooms, smoking but probably not talking much, or loitering aimlessly in the corridors. It is often very difficult to distinguish them from members of staff since the nurses discarded their uniforms during the 1960s, although there has recently been an overdue tendency to frown on jeans and sloppy sandals. However, most of the patients will be elsewhere, involved in some purposeful or purposeless activity. The former include group therapy, interviews with doctors, psychologists, or social workers, or art 'therapy', drama, music, occupational therapy, marital counselling, playing games, or gardening. Many of these institutions used to run their own farms until an enlightened Ministry of Health in the early-1960s decided that involving patients in voluntary agricultural work smacked of slave labour and decreed that it should cease. Now, patients are allowed to follow the healthy, creative pursuits they may well practise in their ordinary lives, as long as the result is decorative rather than useful. The patients have a wide variety of different types of disorder, but to a surprising degree, the same psycho-social therapy package is appropriate to them all. They all have problems socializing, problems with forming and maintaining stable relationships, problems with coping with the world and its inhabitants. Entertaining, or at least receiving, visitors can therefore be regarded as a highly purposeful activity: going into town possibly rather less so, and strolling around the grounds alone is not greatly encouraged.

The psychiatric hospital is divided into three main areas of activity. The acute unit consists of 100 beds, the longer-stay rehabilitation unit has 150, and the psychiatry of old age (a clumsy term, but greatly to be preferred to 'psycho-geriatrics' which combines two debased linguistic coins in one) has a further 150. There is, in addition, a drinking problem unit which has seven beds, and all the units receive varying numbers of day patients who illustrate how much better hospitals can cater for those who happen to live nearby than those in the farther-flung outposts of their empires. There are no fewer than 15 adult psychiatrists, who take it in turn to be on emergency duty to cover the acute unit. Most of them have their own special interest, and much of their work is carried out on an out-patient basis, some of it in fairly distant GP health centres and even in patients' own homes accompanied by the GP. Some of the nurses also go out into the community although based in the hospital. In the present-day jargon, out-reach into the community is very much the flavour of the month. Most of the drinking problem work is community-based with patients attending the hospital if necessary. The consultant in charge would very much like to move his unit into a large house in a suburb of the city. Treatment is aimed at withdrawal more often than 'controlled drinking' which tends not to work.

Another activity which seldom impinges on the wards is the drug dependency clinic which is located in the city and which is a veritable mingling of the disciplines. It is, for administrative purposes, under the titular leadership of a consultant, but is mainly run by the junior medical staff undergoing psychiatric training. A great deal of the day-to-day counselling and follow-up is carried out by the nursing staff and perhaps even more by the social workers. There are probably about 100 addicts on the books at any one time and appointments may be made about every two months. When one of these youngsters (the oldest patient is 39) is first taken on, he is admitted to the ward

for two weeks assessment and a trial of withdrawal. Some patients
become quite ill because they are physically addicted, but more of
them are only psychologically habituated and perhaps have a less
than iron resolve to kick the habit. Those who cannot realistically be
withdrawn altogether are converted onto methadone which is at least
fairly containable and the clinic issues prescriptions every two weeks
or so for a supply of tablets or ampoules for intravenous injection. The
philosophy is to enable the patient to function at a reasonable social
level in terms of holding their jobs, maintaining a stable family
relationship, and avoiding crime. Anyone who commits a drug-
related offence is liable to be struck off the register of attenders. At the
moment, only one patient is maintained on a regular supply of heroin,
and he is always seen by the consultant, who has a special Home
Office licence to authorise this practice.

'What do you feel about these people?' I asked one senior registrar,
a sensible girl, planning a career in general adult psychiatry. Her
reply was a gentle but firm reproach. 'You have to be non-
judgemental in medicine. If you deny help to people with self-induced
disorders, that eliminates all smoking-related diseases, sports injuries,
and traffic accidents for a start. The patients of the DDC need help,
and sometimes they are very rewarding and often they make you
despair. But someone has to do something for them'. Perhaps even
more importantly, someone has to try to learn about them. Another
small subspecialty is the department of child and family psychiatry
which looks after disturbed children and adolescents. It has a few
beds, but does a great deal of out-patient and community work and
liaises extensively with the social services department, the school
health service, educational psychologists, speech therapists, and
teachers.

The acute unit receives six or ten admissions daily, the majority of
GP requests, whatever the exact nature of the disorder, falling into
two categories: disturbed behaviour not containable at home, and
danger of suicide. The diagnostic ranking order of admissions would
be headed by depressive episodes—either true depressive illness or
depression as the dominant feature of some other problem. Then
would come the manic-depressives, whose illness takes the so-called
'bipolar' form of profound depression at one period and a 'high' of
expansive, irrational, equally unmanageable behaviour at another.
Next comes the tragic group of diseases which go under the name of
schizophrenia. Even in this day and age of major tranquillizers, often
given at monthly intervals by depot injection, there remain perhaps 8

per cent of patients who make no response to treatment. Many of these, unless well-supported at home, graduate to the rehabilitation centre where they stay months, years, or forever. The aim of the consultant in charge of the rehabilitation unit is again to get his patients back out in the community. This he is trying to do by the purchase of houses in the city which are run as hostels. To date there are only two, with six and eight patients respectively. This venture is expensive in terms of staff and is unlikely to expand in the foreseeable future, so many of the patients who are discharged to make room for new ones wind up as vagrants or intermittent prisoners.

After these major disorders comes a rag-bag of other conditions which include obsessional states, anxiety and other neuroses, psychopathic and other personality disorders. And in addition to receiving requests from GPs, most of which are handled by the duty registrar, the psychiatrist whose turn it is to be on call can be contacted by the local police and invited to sort out someone who has been picked up as a result of bizarre and deviant behaviour and is now shouting the odds or threatening to kill himself. Similarly, he is on call for the RI who often find themselves with acute psychiatric problems in A&E or on the wards: on one occasion a patient on a medical ward on the fifth floor attacked another patient with a broken bottle prior to throwing himself out of the window. People who become physically unwell due to psychiatric disorder wind up at the RI. This includes patients with septicaemia or hepatitis, or AIDS from self-injection with dirty needles. It also includes a steady stream of more than 10 incidents of self-poisoning a week, some of which require stomach washing, some are comatose and may require ventilation by a respirator, a few require removal of the poison by an artifical kidney. If and when these patients recover, the medical staff usually request an assessment by the psychiatrist who has made a special study of what it is no longer fashionable to describe as 'attempted suicide'. Other patients are brought to A&E by relatives or friends on account of minor episodes of self-poisoning insufficient to render them seriously ill, but possibly indicative of a seriously self-destructive urge. These patients are referred directly to the duty psychiatrist, and some are admitted to the psychiatric hospital for treatment.

The psycho-social aspects of psychiatric hospital treatment have been touched on. What does the doctor do? He interviews each patient admitted in the totally inadequate accommodation set aside for this purpose. A complaint was recently lodged against one of the consultants for interviewing a disturbed patient in the bathroom,

there being no other room available at the time. The junior staff are
expected to make a physical examination: seldom do they embark on
much in the way of laboratory investigations, and the X-ray facilities
on site are just about adequate for the occasional chest film. There is,
incidentally, a sick-bay, but psychiatric nurses are often less than
expert at dealing with physical illness and any patient who becomes at
all seriously sick, unless aged and imminently terminal, is transferred
over to the RI. Contrary to popular belief, few psychiatrists practise
psychotherapy, and only one of ours does so to any formal extent.
Most patients, therefore, receive pills—peace pills, happy pills—and
very effective they often are, too. However, be prepared for another
shock horror exposé: three times a week, some 12 patients are
subjected to electroconvulsive therapy (ECT)—that supposedly most
outrageous of abuses of human rights. This treatment is not only life-
saving in its effects, it has been described as a safer form of treatment
of elderly patients with severe depression than anti-depressant tablets.
It has been calculated that ECT causes one death in 50 000
treatments which is less than deaths from depression (due to suicide
or self-neglect) in patients denied it.

The psychiatrist of old age has an inherently impossible task. It is
to provide a comprehensive service to the elderly in his patch, which
means a considerable case load in terms of depression, anxiety,
alcoholism, and liaison work such as acute confusional states
(delirium) on the medical, geriatric, and surgical wards. It means a
totally overwhelming caseload in terms of senile dementia, that most
pathetic of the ills that ageing flesh is heir to. There are about three-
quarters of a million afflicted in the United Kingdom at the time of
writing, many of whom have no close family, and the consultant's task
is to apologize to relatives, GPs, neighbours, and social workers, that
the Secretary of State has failed to provide him with the tools for the
job. The 'tools', in this context, basically implies resources for
institutional care, since community care for this section of the
population is all too often a euphemism for community neglect. There
being only one consultant, and he being very much involved with
postgraduate education, and also having the power to prescribe for
his demented patients little other than nursing care, a situation has
arisen which applies to many psychiatric hospitals throughout the
country. It is a microcosm of the enduring struggle of the nursing
profession to shrug off the yoke of medical domination. We do the
caring, the nurses clamour, so why should the doctor be the one who
rations it out? Why should we not have the power of admission and

discharge? Because, says the doctor, it is I who in law carries the final overall responsibility for the welfare of the patient. Only I can make a diagnosis and therefore a prognosis. Ultimately, the buck stops here.

Fifteen years ago, the strident demands for greater democracy in our institutions was only a whisper. Until then, the benevolent dictatorship of the medical superintendent reigned supreme especially in the mental hospitals. He had the right to hire and fire, and generally exercised the former, in terms of junior medical staff, according to whether his hospital had greater need of a bowler or a wicket-keeper. The medical superintendents were swept away and replaced by faceless committees of faceless administrators. Now they, too, have been swept away and replaced once more by autocratic managers. The difference between these and the superintendent of yesterday is that these have no qualifications at all and are likely to move on after three or five years (see Chapter 13). It is possibly worthy of note that one of our most successful trading competitors, Japan, remains firmly in the Dark Ages insofar as its treatment of its mentally ill is concerned. Japan's psychiatric services share many of the characteristics of those in the United Kingdom during the 1950s— large numbers of huge, dilapidated hospitals, a vast long-term in-patient population, most of whom are compulsory patients, few obvious attempts to restore independence. Brilliant industrial perfor-mance does not always correlate with humanitarian development— 'we live in a society, not an economy'.

11

High tech:
Radiology, radiotherapy

Many years ago, in the antediluvian era when those of us who are now
senior consultants qualified, the X-ray department was generally an
obscure subterranean region where girls in white uniforms took
pictures which they then respectfully submitted to the scrutiny of the
proper doctors on the wards. The girls were the radiographers, and
we knew that there were also some doctors beavering away down
there who called themselves radiologists, but the physicians and
surgeons of the day treated them with a degree of scorn and declared
that they preferred to look at the films themselves rather than pay any
attention to some so-called doctor who only dealt in shadows rather
than real patients. Thus, the thought of this type of medical career,
lacking the excitement of ultimate responsibility for real patients, did
not have much appeal. However, not having an ongoing responsibility
for the care of patients can become appealing, I am told, especially
after you have enjoyed the privilege of direct patient care for a few
years. Anyway, things have changed a great deal since then, and
radiology has undergone more exciting and dramatic changes than
any other hospital specialty during the past 20 years. The radiologists
are the meek who have inherited the earth, and they are now nothing
like so meek as they used to be. They are the experts who make all the
clever diagnoses with their expensive, complicated machines when the
simple clinicians, with their clumsy, groping fingers have failed. They
are the scientists who understand physics and computers, and how to
purchase vastly expensive pieces of equipment. Increasingly, they are
the doctors who insert needles into deep and distant recesses and who
navigate fine probing tubes down remote, uncharted passages into the
innermost depths of the body. Furthermore, they *know* everybody: the
surgeons, the physicians, the gynaecologists, the paediatricians—even
some of the psychiatrists.

Not that the patient's first encounter with the X-ray department is
glamorous. The chances are that you go for a simple X-ray of your
chest, or a bone, because you have attended the out-patient clinic and

the consultant in charge of your case has suggested these special tests as well as a range of blood samples for various investigations. Alternatively, you have arrived as an emergency and the X-rays come as part of a rather bewildering initiation ceremony designed to test your ability to withstand the psychological stress of containing your discomfort while being taken you know not where, being deserted for you know not how long, and awaiting a decision you know not from who about your personal immediate future. The junior doctors who see you, and the porters who wheel you, and the radiographers who photograph you, seem quite unable to commit themselves in any but the most perfunctory terms concerning what is going to happen to you.

The department is conveniently situated close to the out-patient clinics, near to radiotherapy because the radiotherapists are major users of the service, near to A&E, and near to the neurosciences block for the same reasons, but regrettably remote from the main ward block. It covers a floor space the size of a soccer pitch and extends upwards for a total of four storeys. The ground floor is for the simpler investigations and the upper levels are devoted to more sophisticated techniques. There are five basic X-ray rooms each containing a mere £80K or £90K worth of equipment, and three screening rooms whose contents are nearer the £200K mark. These are for contrast studies in which the organ being examined is filled with a substance which is radio-opaque so that a picture emerges of its outline, and in which the radiologist follows the passage of the contrast on his screen. This enables him to observe any suspicious looking areas which persistently fail to fill with contrast and so might represent malignant growths within the organ. Barium meals, to investigate the gullet, stomach, and upper small intestine, and barium enemas, to investigate the lower bowel, are typical examples. Dye can also be injected into a foot vein, to outline the veins of the legs, and this method is the gold standard for the diagnosis of thrombosis. The 'filling defects' being sought will represent not tumours, but clots of blood which have the evil propensity of detaching in large chunks and travelling up the great abdominal venous trunk (the vena cava) to the heart and then lodging in the outflow and obstructing the circulation. Urography also involves an intravenous injection of contrast, usually into an arm vein, but this particular contrast is filtered from the blood by the kidneys and then outlines the system of ducts which collect the urine from the kidneys and deliver it via the ureters down to the bladder. Injectable contrast media are usually iodine compounds for these have the property of being impenetrable to X-rays. Studies of the gut are carried out with a bland-tasting white suspension of barium sulphate. The taste is only relevant when it is the upper gut which is being studied, and even then is not perhaps of prime importance. (In the United Kingdom it is sometimes felt that the nastier the taste, the more likely a remedy must be to do you good. On the other side of the Channel, many more medicines are given in suppository form. The French, for example, regard the mouth as a delicate instrument for the appreciation of their culinary and vinous delights and not to be sullied by such crudities as medicines: we have been thoughtfully provided with another place for the reception of those.)

Despite the advent of endoscopy (see Chapter 5), the barium meal is very much in evidence for the evaluation of indigestion and of iron-deficient anaemia which is likely to be due to oozing of blood from an ulcer. It remains the investigation of first choice in many centres and there is some controversy about the relative merits of radiography and endoscopy in this situation, although endoscopy is more definitive in acute bleeding. A meal may take half-an-hour and will involve a fair amount of twisting and turning as well as a rather alarmingly rapid tilting of the table into an almost upright position. Nevertheless, it is usually well tolerated by the frail and aged and often yields a firm diagnosis which provides a basis for long-term medication to heal an ulcer or an inflamed gullet. In patients with jaundice due to obstruction of the bile duct, the radiologist may perform an investigation called ERCP in which the endoscope is passed down to the duodenum and the little orifice where the bile duct enters the duodenum is identified. A fine tube is advanced into the bile duct from the tip of the instrument and dye is injected up the bile duct and the duct of the pancreas, and films are taken showing their outlines and depicting the shape of any obstruction. Is it a stone or is it a growth? Or possibly a benign stricture? These are the questions that the pictures may help to answer, and it may even be possible to insert a small tube via the abdominal wall and the ducts within the liver to relieve an inoperable obstruction.

Another floor houses the angiography suite. The main room is rather like an operating theatre because the radiologist has to scrub like a surgeon (see Chapter 6), but the lighting is provided by a series of spots rather than an overhead bank of lights because the X-ray machinery is in the way. The radiologist wears his gown over the heavy leaded protective apron which is obligatory for all those present except the patient. An angiogram, or arteriogram, is an X-ray examination of the arteries, and those most commonly required depict the arteries of the legs. Narrowing of these vessels is common, especially in later life, especially in smokers, especially in men, especially in diabetics. Over 4000 amputations are carried out annually in this country for this condition, which causes a great deal of pain and even loss of life. The purpose of doing an arteriogram is to identify those patients with severe symptoms whose disease is technically suitable for arterial surgery to salvage the limb by linking a good source of blood supply with an accessible run-off point. The radiologist carries out the examination under local anaesthetic and punctures the femoral artery in the groin with a fine cannula which he passes up into the aorta. The contrast is injected into the cannula and serial X-ray films taken as it passes down the legs. More recently, the radiologists have gone further than this: after examining the films, if an accessible and not too extensive atheromatous obstruction is seen, they may proceed to balloon dilatation. A flexible catheter is introduced over a guide-wire until the tip is situated just beyond the obstruction, and a polyvinyl balloon near the tip is forcibly inflated to disperse the atheromatous deposit. The pressure gradient across the obstruction can be measured before and after, and further films can be taken after the procedure, but the immediate change from a cold, blue foot to a warm pink one may offer convincing evidence of success. The technique is not without some discomfort, but it is a whole lot better than major surgery and much less hazardous and the patient is much more quickly up and about afterwards. Particularly for the older, frailer subjects with lungs damaged by years of smoking, it represents a real advance. In 1977, it was first applied to narrowed coronary arteries, and coronary dilatation was introduced at the RI in the early-1980s and is carried out in the cardiac catheterization laboratory with the cardiac surgical team on standby in case of complications. It is performed under local anaesthetic and a degree of sedation. The usual point of access is again the femoral artery at the groin, but the route is a much longer one up the great arterial trunk of the aorta and then down to the mouths of the coronary vessels just as the aorta leaves the heart. The catheter is steered by remote control and it is possible to negotiate the much narrower and more tortuous course of each of the main coronary arteries for much of their lengths. There are, naturally, considerable hazards but the relief of angina is dramatic in successful cases. For obvious reasons, one of the United Kingdom's most skilled radiologists refers to the system as the 'dyno-rod technique'. It is likely that the less crude instrument of the laser beam will be used for this purpose in the foreseeable future.

Angiograms are also used to demonstrate the arteries supplying the brain, usually by direct injection of contrast into the carotid artery in the neck. This is most often done under a general anaesthetic. The films are used by the neurosurgeons in the treatment of certain tumours and in the management of arterial disease threatening a part of the brain or catastrophically pumping a torrent of blood through delicate networks of nerve cells. A recent development known as digital subtraction angiography (DSA) may soon permit adequate views of the arterial system following the injection of contrast into a vein, thereby avoiding the necessity of arterial puncture.

In the bad old days, neurosurgeons used to seek images of tumours within the skull not only by arteriography but also by outlining the brain by the injection of air into the clear fluid in which it is bathed. This unpleasant examination has been rendered obsolete by the introduction of computerized tomography (CT). At the RI we obtained a head scanner in the early-1970s and a body scanner in the early-1980s. Greatly superior images are obtained without the slightest discomfort or hazard to the patient, as long as he or she is able to lie still for 10–20 minutes or sometimes longer. Small children often have to be given a light anaesthetic. The machines look simple and not particularly threatening and embrace the whole patient rather than pointing towards the offending part of the anatomy. At that time, the body scanner cost about £500K. The pictures produced are reconstructed by the computer from information concerning the radiodensity of the body viewed from a large number of directions by a rotating beam of X-rays passing through it from various angles. They represent slices through the body of one to two centimetres thick, and guided by the images on his control and viewing console, the radiologist can needle any structure he wishes, to obtain tissue samples for microscopy or to drain pus from an abscess. The patient lies in reasonable comfort on the table under a great circular gantry, round which the invisible X-ray tube travels with a low humming, buzzing note punctuated by a series of clicks as it engages the selected positions. The time taken to describe this arc over the supine patient is only about two minutes, and the films are then taken away for detailed analysis in the reporting room. The resulting image is exceedingly clear, although it actually consists of a matrix of picture elements (pixels) numbering 240 across and the same up and down, making 57 600 altogether.

There is currently considerable excitement since we have just commissioned a magnetic resonance (MR) imaging apparatus whose

£1 million purchase price was largely raised by public appeal. It has had to be housed in its own new building because of its size and nature. The patient undergoing this type of examination is encased in a huge magnet with a field 10 000 times as strong as that of the earth, which influences the axis of the protons of which he is ultimately constructed which then resonate in response to radio waves. Images are assembled by computer from the emitted radio frequency signals, and these are of even more exquisite quality than those yielded by CT since a slice 1 mm thick is portrayed with a resolution of about 0.33 mm. Moreover, they can be obtained in almost any plane, and without any radiation exposure. Having it done is rather like being slid into a cooker on a baking tray, and is not for the claustrophobic, as it may take as long as 50 minutes, which is a long time even if there is a panic button and soothing music.

The secret of the scanner lies in the magnet which is rendered superconducting by virtually eliminating electrical resistance in the coils by cooling them to -269 °C by means of 750 litres of liquid helium. The magnet presents some problems—it is apt to wipe out the essential strips on any credit cards inadvertently introduced into the machine, and it has been necessary to ensure that the fire extinguishers and resuscitation trolleys in use in the department are constructed of non-magnetic materials. One of the great advantages MR offers over CT lies in its application to the chemical analysis of the tissues being examined, so that, for example, it may prove to be capable of providing critical information concerning the viability of the brains of infants traumatized at birth. Even the straightforward structural pictures are exciting enough—useful information can be obtained, for example, about medium-sized and smallish arteries.

If these technologies appear to be in direct competition with one another, there is yet a third which is in universal use in all X-ray departments and which is simple, cheap and again causes no discomfort or risk, and that is diagnostic ultrasound. The room is an uncluttered one, the operator simply presses a probe against the part he is interested in, and this emits waves of much higher frequency than those audible to the human ear. These are reflected by bone or gas-containing organs but pass through the soft tissues generating echoes where tissues of different physical properties meet. A so-called 'window' will thus permit an uninterrupted path from skin to the structure being studied: objects such as gallstones will cast 'acoustic shadows (or corridors)' behind them. Although less readily interpreted by the untutored eye than CT or MR images, ultrasound pictures are displayed on the TV monitor to the operator who can again use the facility to obtain on-site specimens for subsequent pathological study, whether cells from a tumour or pus from an abscess. The radiologist can pick up abnormalities deep in the liver measuring some one-and-a-half centimetres across by this method, and variations of it produce most valuable information concerning the heart valves and cavities.

There are 40 radiographers at the RI, and 10 radiologists with perhaps 15 junior doctors in training. The department carries out investigations on about 100 in-patients and almost 200 out-patients daily, the substation in the A&E department dealing with about a further 100 cases. All films are kept for seven years at least, and storage is a major commitment and it has been suggested that miniaturization of the films to a 50 mm format may become necessary. The department will do plain chest X-rays and other fairly routine investigations at the request of a GP. Barium meals and enemas can be ordered by the junior hospital doctors, but at the RI, the more invasive or expensive investigations can only be requested by a consultant. The radiologists do like to know why the examination is being requested, as well as by who, and, in addition, whether the patient is fit to undergo what may be quite an arduous procedure and whether he or she is likely to benefit from it. If the radiologist feels that he is being used simply to satisfy the curiosity of the doctor looking after the patient, he may reject the request, usually after a frank and full exchange of views on the telephone.

Nuclear medicine. There is a sign near to the X-ray department bearing the ominous message 'Nuclear Medicine' . . . This is not a sinister preparation for the aftermath of the holocaust, but another high technology specialty geared to probing the abnormal structure and function of the hidden recesses of the human body. The radiologist uses his apparatus to emit radiation which passes through the subject and emerges to imprint shadows on a film. The consultant in nuclear medicine makes the patient emit his own radiation by making him radioactive—or rather, a part of him. He does this by the administration of radioactive compounds which are selectively taken up by certain organs or tissues. He then uses a gamma ray camera to detect this radioactivity and to make pictures of its distribution. These pictures lack the vivid realism of CT studies, but they often give very useful information about the working of an organ as well as, sometimes, its anatomy. The cost in terms of discomfort and danger is very low: in terms of revenue, the department is not one of the RI's big spenders. It produces most of its own radiopharmaceuticals, for instance pertechnetate-labelled sulphur colloid which after injection into a vein is taken up by the liver. 'Cold spots' which will show up in the substance of the liver under the gamma camera may indicate the spread of a cancer arising somewhere distant. An example where nuclear medicine saves lives is the ventilation perfusion lung scan. Radioactive microparticles ranging from 15 to 70 microns in size are injected intravenously and become obstructed in the pulmonary arterioles and capillaries. The gamma camera thus gives a picture of the blood circulation (perfusion) in the lungs. The patient then breathes a mixture of air and a radioisotope of the inert gas krypton from an oxygen mask and an image is obtained of the distribution of air in the lungs (ventilation). The demonstration of parts of the lung which are ventilated but not perfused is strongly suggestive of obstruction in the pulmonary circulation by blood clots, a highly dangerous condition which responds very well to treatment with anticoagulants.

The extension number of the department of nuclear medicine was erroneously given to a panic-stricken public in the aftermath of the Chernobyl reactor disaster. The consultant was far from amused to receive telephone calls from worried ladies whose dogs had been out in the rain and who wondered if it was safe to touch them, and enthusiastic gardeners who had found the tadpoles dying in their fish ponds and who wondered if this was a foretaste of horrors to come. The deluge of calls subsided in a couple of days, but took up a great deal of time while they lasted.

Radiotherapy The cancer doctors refer to their specialty by the rather inelegant term of oncology. They have a considerable empire in terms of patients, manpower, real estate, and plant. There are five of them, and, like the geriatricians and the hospice director, people often ask them whether they do not find their work depressing. All these specialists, on the contrary, seem to be a rather cheery bunch. Perhaps you have to be one of nature's optimists to embark on this kind of career. The oncologists are encamped in one of the larger foothills of the mountain range, a two-storey block protruding out to one side with its own entrance and reception area. It is sometimes called the radiotherapy department (RTD) and was originally intended to serve the whole region, although now two other DGHs have their own departments. Nevertheless, patients come to the RI for cancer treatment from far and wide and 180 radiotherapy treatments arc given every day, and the large majority of these are on an out-patient basis. It should be emphasized that the oncologists do not have a monopoly of cancer by any means. The majority is perhaps to be found in the general surgical and medical units and in the geriatric wards, and there are blood malignancies such as leukaemia which are usually the province of the haematologists. Clinics are held daily in the RTD, and the consultant decides whether radiotherapy is likely to be worthwhile in terms of curing the disease, helping the surgeon to cure it, delaying its progress, or relieving symptoms. With the aid of a computer he will then draw up a plan of treatment based on the image of the growth which he obtains from a CT examination. This plan is translated into radiation doses, duration, direction, and type in such a way that the beam is concentrated on the tumour and as far as possible avoids nearby vital structures which could be seriously damaged. The target zone may be mapped out on the skin, and for some cancers a cast is taken from which a shield is constructed either to protect surrounding tissues or to assist in directing the irradiation. A series of treatments is then scheduled each lasting two to ten minutes or so and occurring perhaps five days a week for three or four weeks.

The treatment area of the RTD is rather a pleasant place, about the size of an indoor tennis court and decorated in a restful bluish-green. It is of an open plan construction and out of office hours it has a spacious air about it. During treatment periods, which are weekday mornings and afternoons, the tranquillity is shattered by the endless comings and goings of people in suits, people in dressing gowns, people in wheelchairs, people on trolleys, and people in beds. Most of the people are patients and their relatives, but here and there a pair of white-uniformed girls in their twenties can be seen sitting at an instrument panel or escorting a patient in or out of a treatment bay. These are the therapeutic radiographers, of which there are about 20, who shine the rays, to distinguish them from diagnostic radiographers, who take the pictures. The treatment bay is round a couple of corners so that the patients are never shut away with the machine. The walls of the bays are a metre thick and made of hardened concrete. Inside is a dimly lit area the size of a living room, with a couch which can be adjusted in any plane. Four of the machines are linear accelerators and after you have been carefully positioned by the radiographers, it is either directed straight at the growth, or if it is deeply situated, it will gradually, and silently, swing over you three to four times to focus the maximum dose on the growth rather than on the skin and other nearby structures. The radiographers depart and sit outside, where they operate the machinery. They are in constant visual contact with the patient, both through a dim, greenish, water-filled porthole in the wall, and by means of a TV screen. However, patients are wonderfully tolerant, especially those with serious illnesses, and nearly all of them lie still and quiet while the great steel girder with its blind cylindrical head inches soundlessly past on its relentless arc.

The department of oncology has one professor and four NHS consultants, and they travel extensively to see patients in other hospitals in the region. They have beds at the RI and are in considerable demand by other departments who have patients with malignant disease. Usually it is necessary to obtain a small sample of tissue by means of a needle biopsy to determine the exact nature of the malignancy, for not all tumours are radiosensitive. Some respond better to drug treatment, especially some forms of widespread tumours of the lymphatic system, and this is another part of the oncologist's work. The drugs are highly toxic, as is radiotherapy—in Hamlet's words 'diseases desperate grown, by desperate appliance are relieved, or not at all'.

There is some concern at the moment because the doctors and nurses who draw the drugs up from the ampoule into the syringe, may inhale minute quantities of the vapour or otherwise come into contact with these very toxic chemicals which could affect the bone marrow or even cause cancers or malformations of babies subsequently borne to them. If you follow a cart down the corridor with the message 'cytotoxic waste' give it a wide berth. It contains syringes, needles, ampoules and bottles contaminated with these drugs on their way to be incinerated at 1000 °C. Another cause for concern for the safety of visiting relatives, other patients, and staff is the technique of treating cancer of the womb by insertion of a radioactive implant. These patients should really be screened-off from contacts, but perfect screening is not practical—not in the crowded, busy wards of the RI.

The commonest cancers on our books are lung, followed by skin, breast, and colon. Many patients are cured, and most are relieved of distressing symptoms. Others are offered meticulous attention to detail in the relief of mental and physical distress of both patient and family in the more tranquil environment of the terminal care hospice in its pleasant surroundings on the western fringe of the city.

Medical physics. Sandwiched between X-ray and radiotherapy is a substantial two-storey annexe which is totally unfamiliar to patients,

nurses, and all too many of the doctors. It houses the Department of
Medical Physics, and the name perhaps acts as something of a
deterrent to many doctors who look back with abhorrence at the hours
they spent measuring electrical resistances, specific gravities, and
grappling with the mysteries of heat and light. All large DGHs will
boast a department of physics, but teaching hospitals tend to have
much bigger ones who undertake a great deal of work for other
hospitals throughout the Region.

Much of the work of the physicists is closely allied to their next door
neighbours. They select and service radiotherapy equipment and the
computers used in planning treatment, and they prepare radioactive
implants used in the treatment of gynaecological and other cancers.
They advise nuclear medicine how to handle radioactive materials
and they have developed suitable protocols for data analysis using
computer processing. They are responsible for the protection of staff
exposed to radiation, particularly the radiologists and radiographers.
One of the many aspects of this is the film badge service which
provides all personnel at risk with little plastic badges to be worn on
the white coat to record the level of radiation received. The dose is
recorded on micro-computer, and about 1500 badges are dealt with
monthly. However, the badges also come from all over the Region as
well as from the private sector, for example dental and veterinary
surgeons using X-ray equipment. A charge of £1.10 is made per film.
The films develop a shade of grey which gives a cumulative dose
measurement, but following the Chernobyl catastrophe they came out
in a rash of readily identifiable spots.

There is a large and well-equipped workshop which constructs
'one-off' pieces of apparatus to order. There is an instrument repair
department which checks blood pressure machines (40 a month) and
sharpens surgical instruments (500 a month). There is a support
workshop which repairs and maintains anaesthetic systems (60 of
them), oxygen flow meters (600), ventilators (100), and a host of other
items. Then there is a clinical measurements section which provides
back-up for all invasive monitoring in theatres and ITU, as well as
studies of blood flow and bladder pressure among others. One
development here has been blood sugar monitoring of diabetic
expectant mothers by telemetry. The computer in the department
produces a print-out in the form of a graph from the six readings taken
daily in the patient's own home, and the medical staff of the diabetic
clinic phone instructions through to ensure tight control. The fetal
heart rate can be monitored by telemetry in the same way. There is

also general computing and information technology, laser safety and maintenance, servicing of dialysis machines, and a flourishing (finance permitting) research programme.

Finally, there is the electronics section, responsible for the care of about 4000 items of equipment with a replacement value of £5 million. At any given time a quantity of this range of hard-ware is therefore to be seen in the department, which is also littered with its own instruments for checking other instruments as well as a useful range of tools and gadgets. Security is a problem—many of these bits and pieces are eminently portable. Crown property is never insured, and in any case the premiums would be too high, so that any theft is a write-off. All this loss, maintenance, and depreciation is an expensive business. The life expectancy of the toys also seems to be declining, in contrast to that of their users: it might have been 10 years, about ten years ago. Today, it is probably nearer five years. Equipment is evolving so rapidly that a spare part for an instrument manufactured today will not be obtainable in five years' time, because the instrument has become a museum piece.

So much for the things: what about the people? There are 10 physicists, all of whom will be graduates and some of whom also hold a PhD or an MSc. The chief physicist is an honorary member of the medical consultant staff. There are about 40–50 medical physics technicians, who probably left school at 16 or 18 and who then entered the department and underwent an apprenticeship and who have since become highly skilled practical craftsmen. Finally, there are a few (far too few) supporting staff such as secretaries and clerks. The physicists are faintly reminiscent of the heroes of Nevil Shute's novels. They are the back-room boffins, crucial to the war effort against the forces of disease and disability, highly skilled and committed, and yet enjoying little of the spotlight of public acclaim.

12

Corpses and corpuscles:
The laboratories

Hospital doctors in Western countries are spoiled. Their colleagues in general practice, and those practising in the developing countries, have to rely heavily on the diagnostic skills of their ears, eyes, and fingers, often deployed under highly adverse conditions. We, at the RI, and at places like the RI, can examine the patient under ideal circumstances, well illuminated, disrobed, hosed down (as is occasionally necessary), displayed on a convenient couch or bed, attended by the nursing staff, and previously or subsequently re-examined by our colleagues. We certainly ought to get it right. However, the main reason we usually get it right eventually is that we are supported by the diagnostic service departments which comprise radiology, or imaging (see Chapter 11) and the laboratories. Virtually all the patients who attend the hospital's clinics or are admitted to its wards undergo various tests. The majority have X-rays, blood tests, or have urine specimens, swabs or sputum samples taken. The blood samples are taken by doctors, students, or occasionally nurses, but there are also a few 'phlebotomists' whose job it is to take the routine specimens. The two or three who work in the out-patient clinics extract 3500 blood specimens from 900 patients a week. The laboratories are absolutely central to the whole function of the hospital and have indeed become totally taken for granted as a highly influential sphere of activity. They occupy a six-storey block and are served by a mechanical delivery system whereby specimens arrive in pint-sized containers catapulted around a network of tubes reminiscent of department stores a few decades ago. They are staffed by doctors, clerks, secretaries, couriers, and by a breed of personnel whom we have yet to meet. These are the medical laboratory scientific officers (MLSOs), and there are about 100 of them at the RI. They are like the rest of the world in being both male and female in roughly equal proportions and they are taken on with two 'A'-levels or, increasingly, with a degree. The latter, if relevant in content, reduces by a year or so the five years required to achieve the final accolade of

Fellow of the Institute of Medical Laboratory Scientists (FIMLS). The pay, initially, is fairly meagre, and there are evening classes and eventually practicals and lectures held in the hospital and examinations to be taken annually. Not so long ago, it was necessary to qualify in more than one of the sciences, but the inexorable trend towards earlier specialization has resulted in the production of MLSOs fully competent in only a single branch of medical science.

The top floor is occupied by haematology; the main laboratory, like those below it, occupies about the space of a tennis court without the surrounds. Every day, 400–500 little pink bottles containing 2.5 ml of blood arrive by courier or through the tube to have a blood count. About 15 per cent are sent by the local GPs, the rest are generated by the hospital clinics and wards. The amount of haemoglobin, the size of the red cells, and the number of white cells and platelets are measured automatically by a machine which accepts the specimen, dilutes it, sends it flowing round a system of diminutive tubes and vessels and eventually produces a computer print-out with the relevant values. This piece of apparatus can handle about 900 blood counts an hour, so there will be little spare capacity until we are forced to invest in a back-up at a cost of £80K. Before each specimen is handed to the machine, one of the MLSOs makes a film on a microscope slide. If any of the values fall outside an acceptable range set by the consultant, the slide is examined under the microscope for a fuller analysis, one MLSO being able to look at about 55 slides in a day. The normal slides are kept for six or eight months, the abnormals which have been examined are stored for eight years. At the time of writing the charge levied for a private blood count is £7 but no one is sure whether this really reflects the life of the machinery as well as staff and materials.

The clotting mechanism of the blood is the province of the haematologists. The main reason for it to become defective is that the doctors have decided that a patient requires anticoagulants. Every day, around 15 blood samples arrive from the wards, and twice a week about 90 from the anticoagulant clinic to be tested and the dose of Warfarin (yes, the rat poison) adjusted so that the blood does not clot in the patient's legs, lungs, arteries, but neither does he bleed spontaneously into his gut, bladder, or muscles. In addition, there are the bleeders, mostly with haemophilia (we look after 50 or so) but a smaller number with Christmas disease, named after the family first identified with it rather than any association with excessive revelry. These patients require regular intravenous injections of blood products to replace the missing clotting factors, sometimes thrice weekly, sometimes only once a fortnight, to stop them bleeding into joints or muscles, or from trivial injuries. Those requiring frequent injections are taught to do it themselves with the help of a relative and call in at intervals to collect their 'groceries'. This group of patients, already having drawn a somewhat short straw, have now become afflicted by the shadow cast by AIDS because a number of those who received treatment before all blood donors were tested now harbour the virus.

Eighty tubes of blood arrive daily in the haematology lab for blood grouping and cross-matching—and often a few more at night for emergency transfusion. A certain amount of blood is kept in stock for each group, and compatability has to be established with the blood of the recipient who has bled from an ulcer, or is undergoing major surgery, or has lost blood in a motor smash, or is seriously anaemic. The cross-matched blood is scrupulously labelled and placed in another refrigerator to await collection. However foolproof the precautions, administration of the wrong blood, sometimes with tragic results, remains a remote hazard of hospitalization. Avoidance depends on rigorous observation of the prescribed drill. The Regional Transfusion Centre, it should be added, is separately housed on the campus of the RI, and is again a sizeable enterprize whose details are perhaps beyond the scope of this book. It organizes the annual collection of 90 000 units, each of 500 ml from our donors who represent about 40 per 1000 of the population. At least 70 000 units are used, 40 000 units being consumed by the RI. At any one time there will be 1200 units in stock, and they are kept for four weeks or so before being turned over to the purification of various derivatives required for clotting disorders or deficiences of other blood derivatives. Whole blood, in fact, is nowadays seldom on offer. The smart, navy-blue vans of the Transfusion Service are a familiar sight on the local motorways.

There is a battery of less frequently requested investigations carried out by haematology. Perhaps 400 specimens of bone marrow, sucked out of the breast bone under local anaesthetic, are examined annually to look for abnormalities in the formation of the blood cells. Most of these are probably from the leukaemia unit which is discussed in Chapter 5.

One floor down from the haematologists dwell the biochemists (or chemical pathologists) who run a similar scale of operation with an annual budget of £500K. Two-thirds of this goes in salaries for the 25

MLSOs, 10 biochemists, and five doctors, who are presided over by the genial figure of the professor. The MLSOs never reach a salary much in excess of about £16K including overtime, even though it is an increasingly graduate profession. The biochemists are likely to have a Ph.D., and will ultimately achieve a salary of approximately £20K. Unlike the duty MLSO in haematology who has to sleep in because of the likelihood of an urgent cross-match during the night, the MLSO on duty for biochemistry can go home provided it is nearby, although there is a very high probability of several calls during the night.

Most of the biochemical tests are carried out on blood samples. Half of this workload consists of requests for the blood urea, which is a breakdown product of protein and a guide to the function of the kidneys, and the electrolytes—sodium, potassium, chloride, and bicarbonate, which if significantly abnormal can indicate a profound disturbance of the body's chemical balance. Together with these the same sample yields a blood sugar level, although if a highly accurate estimation is required a separate sample is required. However, the so-called 'screen' gives a good idea whether the patient is diabetic, and if known to be, whether the disease is reasonably well controlled. The set of information from this 5 ml plastic tube of anticoagulated blood, the urea and electrolytes, is termed the U&Es, or, in some countries, the ionogram. Probably, the next commonest battery of investigations are the liver function tests (LFTs) which indicate whether the liver is capable of excreting the bile pigment, which is derived from the haemoglobin in the old, broken-down red cells (each has a life-span of about 100 days). If not, whether this is due to destruction of liver cells or obstruction to the bile duct down which the bile flows into the gut. The LFTs also indicate the amount of calcium in the blood, which may be abnormal in a number of bone and metabolic disease states. Then there are various enzymes which are measured in the blood as an indication that they have been leaked out of damaged cells, for example heart muscle cells injured by a coronary thrombosis. The blood proteins are often of importance and are quantified in the LFTs but analysed more closely in certain situations. There are the blood gases (oxygen and carbon dioxide) which require arterial rather than venous blood. The former is taken by the houseman, the latter by houseman, student, or the ladies in white coats ('phlebotomists') whose job it is to visit the wards and clinics doing just that. The blood gases are affected by serious lung disease leading to respiratory failure and are repeatedly measured in patients in ITU. There are also the endocrine investigations which measure, for instance, the amount of circulating thyroxine and thus whether the thyroid gland is over-active or under-active. A rapidly expanding field is 'therapeutic drug monitoring'. If an epileptic continues to have fits despite being prescribed an anticonvulsant, an adequate blood level of the drug suggests he needs to change to a different anticonvulsant, an inadequate level suggests he needs a larger dose, and a zero reading suggests he is not taking his tablets.

All these are fairly routine investigations in the United Kingdom and are highly automated and computerized. The main laboratory has an area set aside with a bench full of miniature machines to process single specimens which are urgent such as blood sugars in diabetics in coma. However, usually they are done on large machines which accept a batch at a time. Some are boxes which give no clue as to what is going on inside them but merely spew out information on the inevitable VDU accompanied by the inevitable computer print-out. The U&E machine is a cheerful piece of apparatus, the size of a refrigerator, which has a visible network of fine pipettes and tubing containing coloured reagents and you can see it busily diluting, adding, and transferring them from one vessel to another. It handles 90 samples an hour but its capacity will soon be exceeded. It cost £20K in 1977 but a bigger, better replacement with added facilities will be nearer £500K.

Some chemical analyses are carried out on bodily material other than blood. Quite a quantity of urine arrives daily for U&E estimation, and for identification of obscure metabolites in rare diseases. In the corner stands a large fume cupboard, because one of the less satisfying tasks of the department of chemical pathology is the detection of traces of blood in the stools of patients who are anaemic and may have a lesion oozing miniscule quantities of blood hidden somewhere in the gut. An even less pleasant request is the measurement of the amount of fat in the faeces collected over a three-day period to establish whether there is a failure of fat absorption due to intestinal or pancreatic disease.

Many of the samples received, therefore, yield a reading of several different measurements. The number of figures sent by the department to the clinicians for perusal and filing in the case notes is now about a million a year, performed on about 150 000 specimens. Perhaps 15 per cent of the workload comes from general practice, 5 per cent from the organ transplantation programme, and the remaining 80 per cent emanates from the wards and the out-patient clinics. An annual revenue of £10K is generated by the private hospital and by carrying out tests at the behest of a pharmaceutical company whose product is undergoing a clinical trial and who is anxious to detect any liver damage, for example, that it might cause. The charge for these investigations is £7 per test, but the figure is one which was conjured up out of thin air rather than one which reflects accurate assessment.

The biochemists have voiced two main concerns of late. One is the remorseless, exponential increase in the demands made upon them. This stems from two factors, one of which is the steadily increasing activity of virtually all departments of the hospital in the absence of any real increase in its funding. The other reason is the somewhat profligate use of investigations by junior medical staff who tend to carry out a routine battery of baseline investigations (the 'pan-scan' or 'poly-investogram') on every patient admitted, fearing, all too often correctly, that the chief is more likely to pass adverse comments during his rounds on errors of omission than those of commission. The argument is that many diseases, especially in the frail elderly, can be insidious and difficult to diagnose and yet treatment may be very worthwhile. The problem is that there is little hard evidence as to how worthwhile, or which diseases, and consequently which tests should be done on a 'screening' basis—that is, without being triggered by some clinical pointer to a likely diagnosis.

The other development which is causing both concern and excitement is the evolution of bedside, or consulting room, bio-chemistry. Desk-top machines are becoming available on the Con-tinent whereby the clinician can obtain readings of his patients' glucose, electrolyte, and blood cholesterol levels within a minute or two. The glucometer has been available in hospital wards for over 10 years, and many diabetics now possess their own. The disadvantage of such undoubtedly advantageous techniques is that, on the whole, it is easier to obtain a seriously erroneous reading than an accurate one, and neither user nor apparatus are subject to the quality control built into the system in a first-class laboratory such as that at the RI.

So far, the biochemists are not greatly disturbed by AIDS: the design of the specimen bottles minimizes the need for handling, and high-risk specimens receive individual treatment. Should the number escalate, they warn, their current regular budgeting overspend will appear insignificant because of the implications for increasing staff and plant.

One flight of stairs, or, if you have time to spare, a single lift-stop down, brings you to the upper of the two floors devoted to virology, immunology, and, bigger than either of those, bacteriology—or microbiology, as it prefers to be called. This is on a similar scale to haematology and chemical pathology, although some of the personnel and some of the bench space is occupied by a national organization outside the jurisdiction of the RI—the Public Health Laboratory Service, which maintains a nation-wide surveillance of infectious diseases. However, the department functions smoothly enough as a single unit and fulfils certain vital roles in the hospital such as the continuous provision of control of infection guidance and taking the lead in the formulation of antibiotic policy. The number of specimens received each year is now 160 000 (45 per cent from GPs) and is increasing steadily. The nature of these specimens is aesthetically unedifying. It includes a greenish version of salad cream which is coughed up by the large number of patients with acute infective exacerbations of their chronic cigarette-induced lung disease; mal-odorous samples of urine from those unfortunate enough to have a catheter, or to have a urinary tract infection (UTI) for any other reason. It includes fresh stools from patients with diarrhoea; swabs from festering sores on buttocks, heels and legs, and operation wounds; vast numbers of throat swabs from general practitioners faced with coughs and colds and sore throats of epidemic proportions. All sorts of other samples are sent to the laboratory: cerebrospinal fluid, in cases where meningitis or cerebral abscess or encephalitis is suspected; blood cultures when there is nothing direct to send because most infections cause a low grade septicaemia from time to time and some illnesses are predominantly septicaemic from the word go. Infections are a very common cause of admission to the medical and geriatric wards, and a frequent and greatly feared complication on the surgical wards. The various specimens are therefore examined microscopically without delay and plated-out into various delicious culture media consisting of broths and jellies full of succulent nutrients to await the growth of little furry islands of bacterial colonization. Identification of the bacterial species is not enough, because the next step is treatment, thus the sensitivity of the organism to the range of current antimicrobials needs to be determined. The microbes are constantly developing resistance to the therapeutic armamentarium and the drug manufacturers are constantly developing new generations of antibiotic, thus the bacteriologists are assured of a secure and varied future.

Symbolically located below ground level, at the bottom of the laboratory block, is an empire which is all too familiar to most of the clinicians and which is officially, and rather archaically, designated 'department of morbid anatomy'. Within this empire are five interdependent territories—the mortuary, the post-mortem room, the histology and pathology labs, the chapel of rest, and the coroner's office. The emperor is untouched by the macabre nature of his domain and is an exuberant, aggressive professor of considerable eminence, who unreservedly claims the title of head of department and exercises a (usually) benevolent dictatorship over the six NHS consultants as well as the similar number of juniors.

The mortuary can accommodate 54 occupants but does not pride itself on a high occupancy and at any one time may perhaps hold six or 10 bodies at a temperature of 4 °C. Not all come from the wards, of course. There is a steady trickle of BIDs (brought in dead, usually traffic victims or coronaries) from A&E as well as all other sudden, accidental, or suspicious deaths from the community because these come under the jurisdiction of the coroner who will order an autopsy to be carried out and who will, if he feels that further clarification is necessary, arrange for an inquest to be held. Many of the deaths occurring in the wards of the RI also have to be reported to the coroner, including all those where an accident or a medical mishap or alcohol or a drug contributed to the death or where death has occurred so soon after admission that it may not have been possible to arrive at a diagnosis.

Even if the coroner has not become involved, the professor of pathology likes to have as many deaths submitted to post-mortem examination as possible, and so do most of the clinicians. It is policy, therefore, at the RI, that every time an aged and failing patient eventually succumbs to an entirely natural and commonplace illness, the house officer approaches the grieving family to request their permission for it to be carried out. This is on two grounds—to be certain that everything possible has been done, and to submit ourselves to audit and widen our knowledge base. Some of the house officers balk at this task, and many relatives refuse, characteristically, totally illogically, but totally understandably on the irrefutable grounds 'he/she has been through enough already'. An educated guess would be that 20 per cent of those deaths not referred to the coroner come to autopsy, and a rather more reliable statistic is that 900 necropsies are performed annually, of which about half are coroner's cases. Each working morning, therefore, three or four naked corpses lie on the gleaming slabs equipped with hoses, sponges, bowls, and knives, awaiting the duty pathologists. The examination probably takes about an hour, and is conducted with meticulous respect. The external appearance is particularly important in forensic work, less so in hospital cases. In the latter, it is the internal organs which are of interest and these are removed through a long incision from the pelvis to the neck. Individual organs are inspected and weighed: tubes such as the intestine, the windpipe, the bile duct, the coronary arteries, followed and opened through their length. Abscesses, tumours, blood clots, haemorrhages, deformed heart valves will be noted and anything unusual discussed with colleagues from neighbouring tables. Do the pathologists' findings explain the death and tally with the diagnosis arrived at during life, or have obvious clues been missed? The post-mortem room has long been regarded as medicine's 'court of final appeal'. The consultants formerly in charge of the patient's case or his juniors will try to arrive in time to be shown the abnormalities and discuss them with the wisdom of hindsight—that most effective of diagnostic instruments, the 'retrospectoscope'. Sometimes, the clinicians have got it wrong: not infrequently, a final unexpected collapse has not been correctly diagnosed: but most often, the principal pathologies have been well defined prior to death. Not surprisingly, in view of the advanced age of most deceased patients, it is quite common to find lesions, particularly tumours, which were unsuspected during life because they are early and small and have not yet made themselves felt and were unrelated to the main illness. It is also quite usual to find nothing which adequately explains the patient's demise, not because 'old age' is now regarded as a respectable cause of death but because so many deaths are due to disturbances of function rather than of structure. Abnormalities of the rhythm of the heart may be such as to effectively halt the circulation, and disturbances of the chemical constitution of the blood may be incompatible with life. Any particularly dramatic specimens will be photographed and perhaps demonstrated to the students during the lunch hour. Samples of the various tissues are taken for subsequent microscopic examination which may be the only means of determining, for example, the type of kidney disease or the origin of a widespread cancer that has been found to have invaded the liver, lungs, and lymph nodes. Finally, the organs are returned to the body and one of the mortuary attendants will skilfully stitch the incision and carefully clean up so that, once the shroud is replaced, the body looks peaceful and undamaged. This is true even when it has been necessary to examine the brain, since the skull vault and scalp are replaced with consummate care.

I only recall one occasion on which a body was treated with less than scrupulous respect, when it happened to be that of a distinguished foreigner. The pathologist was interrupted by an urgent knock on the door to notify him that the hearse had arrived to take the remains to a waiting aircraft for transportation home. Having far from finished with the internal organs he hurriedly grabbed a set of spares from the next table, put them in and closed up. The sequel was embarrassing. On arrival at destination, the receiving medical authorities deemed it prudent to conduct their own post-mortem, and were quite unable to identify the evidence on which the professor had based his reported findings.

Our department holds regular 'clinico-pathological conferences' with the pathologists to go through cases of special interest or those which have caused a great deal of worry or doubt. The pathologist who conducted the autopsy demonstrates the tissues under a microscope which transfers the image onto a large television screen. These sessions provide valuable teaching for both sides but tend to take place several weeks after the death because the histology laboratory is under considerable pressure and naturally has to give priority to tissue samples taken from the living, either at operation or by means of a biopsy in the ward or X-ray department. Approximately 12 000 surgical specimens come into the laboratory annually, and there is a considerably greater workload of 30 000 cytological smears. These consist of sputum, to search for tell-tale cells from a lung cancer, smears from the neck of the womb for the same purpose, urine, fluid from chest or abdomen or anywhere that might have malignant cells shed into it, because the technique does not involve a surgical operation. The pathologists, like everyone else, tend to specialize. Two of them carry out the bulk of the forensic work and are liable to be called out to examine corpses discovered in the rich variety of scenarios that mankind's evil genius is capable of devising, before having them transported back to the clinical sterility of the ivory tower. They enjoy this work, apparently: an illustration of the truth of the overworked cliché that it is a good thing that we are not all born alike. The professor was appointed to his Chair about 30 years ago, when the three counties of our Region managed to offer him a couple of homicides a year to investigate. He now has to confine his forensic work to our own county where the homicide rate has now risen to almost one a week.

13

Take me to your leader: Management

It has often been commented that a little green alien who landed his flying saucer in the grounds of an NHS hospital and issued the standard request in fluent English to be taken to our leader would be greeted with total incomprehension. Who is the leader in such a democratic organization? The chairman of the Health Authority? The senior member of the management? The senior physician or surgeon, or nurse? Who runs the hospital? The question is ridiculous: it is a team effort. Such, at least, has been the received wisdom in many quarters for many years, until the current turmoil which has shattered this cosy, if rather vague perception.

Perhaps it is worth briefly recapitulating the structure of the hospital service during the past two decades. During the 1960s and early-1970s, the teaching hospitals still had their Boards of Governors who employed a House Governor and gave him a great deal of authority. Other hospitals were grouped under Hospital Management Committees (HMCs) which were in turn grouped into the various Regions (14 in England) with their Regional Hospital Boards (RHBs). Some of the individual non-teaching hospitals, particularly establishments such as the psychiatric hospitals and the sanatoria where patients had been likely to be resident for periods of months or even years during the 1950s, but also some of the general hospitals had a medical superintendent. He was a member of the consultant staff and no one in such a hospital would have had the slightest hesitation in conducting the visiting alien straight to his august presence.

Sir Keith Joseph, the then Secretary of State, inspired by a firm of management consultants, changed all that in 1974 with the first reorganization. The RHBs became Regional Health Authorities (RHAs). The HMCs were demolished and so were most of the Boards of Governors. In came concensus management: Area Health Authorities would correspond with the recently re-drawn county boundaries and would have an appointed chairman and members representing local government, the trades unions, the local university, and the healthcare professions. Each Area contained two or three Districts which might be centred on a sizeable town and would boast a DGH with a catchment population of approximately a quarter of a million citizens. The upheaval of the 1974 reorganization achieved little in the way of visible improvements and spawned a proliferation of committees and bureaucracy. A further tinkering with the mechanics during the 1980s, again by a Conservative administration, swept away the totally redundant Area tier but few of the administrators, most of whom found niches elsewhere in the service. In the event, very few heads rolled. The RHAs retained their large office blocks and their teams of officers: Health Authority members being amateurs, they needed the advice of the professionals so there was a Regional Medical Officer (largely administrative), a Regional Nursing Officer, an Administrator, and a Treasurer. The Districts became much more autonomous and those like ourselves with a teaching hospital were dignified by a 'T' after their names. The District Health Authority had its team of officers and there was also a District Management Team (DMT) in which the officers were supplemented by a consultant and a general practitioner. The general practitioners, it should be noted, continued to remain independent contractors and not employees of the NHS, but the Health Authority ran those Health Centres where the premises were not the property of the GPs as well as running community nursing, the schools medical service, health education for the public, chiropody, and public health. The powerful figure of the County Medical Officer of Health had left the stage in 1974.

Under the DMT were a number of units run each by a Unit Management Group of Consultant, Nurse, and Administrator and they might represent acute hospital services, psychiatric services, care of the elderly, midwifery and children, and the community. Everything was run by groups, teams, or committees. Until Mr Roy Griffiths, managing director of Sainsbury's, was commissioned by Mrs Thatcher's government to lead an inquiry into management arrangements in the NHS and made his report public in October 1983. The next two years saw the far-reaching recommendations of that report being implemented at speeds ranging from unseemly haste to frank foot-dragging throughout the 191 Health Districts (in England—there are several more in the other countries) by a government which had long been irritated by its apparent inability to control what it saw as a bottomless pit of waste and inefficiency. One of the recommendations which has been totally circumvented by a devious civil service concerned the DHSS, occupying vast London office blocks at the Elephant and Castle and Euston. The Elephant was to become trimmer and leaner, more of a racehorse perhaps, and drastically curb its massive output of paper, much of it of minimal importance, which it sends to Regions and Districts. This has signally failed to happen. At local level, however, a new breed of fixed-contract managers, many of them from industry or commerce and with no knowledge of health services whatever, have replaced the anonymous administrators and many of the officers too. People who thought that they were totally secure found that their jobs had disappeared almost overnight. Administrators, nursing officers, treasurers, suddenly found that the District General Manager (or Chief Executive) had decided that he could manage perfectly well without them. All the way down the line people felt vulnerable and insecure, and morale sagged.

It is too early to say whether these changes will turn out to be good or bad. If management means that an identifiable person is entrusted with sufficient responsibility to take decisions instead of the frustrating, endless referral from one committee to another, that must be good. (Getting shelves put up in a store cupboard can take months.) At the RI the top job has gone, not to a health service professional, but to the sort of animal the government had in mind, with a background in business and local government. Although he arguably has greater power to spoil the service than to improve it, he has certainly grasped the essential nettles with commendable energy— after all, his own (£45K a year) job depends upon it. Our problems are mainly due to inadequate finance: we are looking at ways of generating some ourselves since the government certainly will not give us more. The incinerator now earns us £35K a year by destroying documents and other rubbish from outside the NHS, and contributes to heating the hospital. Our Chief Executive is determined to put the infrastructure right—switchboard, portering, secretarial services— without which the shining image of the emporium of high technology healing so easily becomes tarnished. Nevertheless, it is undoubtedly hard that many people who joined the NHS thinking it offered tenure for life should find that the rules have suddenly been re-written, however laudable the underlying philosophy.

Now that the 'management' bandwagon has gathered momentum, it will soon be time to take stock and ask 'Is your hospital well managed?' It may not be possible to reply with a straight yes or no, but there are a few simple guidelines which might help patients and staff to decide for themselves. If the place is well run, I suggest that:

(a) There should not be a waiting period of more than a few weeks for an out-patient appointment.

(b) Patients should not have to wait a long time in out-patients.

(c) There should not be a waiting period of more than a few weeks for admission for 'routine' surgery.

(d) Patients should receive reasonable notice of their admission—perhaps a month or so: the longer the wait, the more unreasonable does an immediate summons appear to be.

(e) There should be easy communication by 'phone.

(f) Delays due to lack of porters should be unknown.

(g) Patients should not spend any time in hospital with nothing happening (unless too sick to be at home).

(h) There should not be delays in discharge because of a lack of simple aids, e.g. wheelchairs, commodes, social support.

(i) Staff vacancies should be promptly filled.

(j) The staff is loyal and stays in post.

(k) The place and its staff should look neat and clean, and all staff should be helpful.

(l) The facilities should be used maximally.

(m) Wastage should be minimal.

The consultants, it must be said, would certainly not regard the general manager as our leader. He is there as an enabler, they would say. Patients come to hospital to see and be treated by doctors, and all else is subservient to that central activity, and the manager is there to ensure that the consultants have the staff, the equipment, and the facilities with which to treat their patients. So who is *their* leader? The professor of medicine? The senior physician? The dean of the medical school? Their representative on the District Management Board? Or the Health Authority? Perhaps, at the RI it is none of these august persons, but the Chairman of the Consultant Staff. It is his task to offer the corporate professional view of his colleagues to the Authority on every aspect of the running of the hospital service locally—an inherently impossible task, but a vital one nevertheless since the service cannot function without medical advice and co-operation.

Of the other personnel with a claim to be the leader, the nurses have to a large extent been displaced by the latest restructuring (see Chapter 3). Perhaps the Chairman of the Health Authority has the strongest claim: the manager is, after all, the hired employee of the Authority and so, for that matter, in a Teaching District, are the medical staff. The Chairman is appointed by the government and it is a part-time post for which he is thought to be paid a salary of £12K a year. Being the Chairman involves him in a great deal more than simply chairing the meetings, although that in itself is an unenviable task. The 19 members of the Authority meet monthly, the meetings last for several hours, and having seen the papers I can readily believe the assurances I have received that they are unutterably tiresome. They are often padded out with a great deal of trivia, some of the discussion is frankly political, and the local press hovers hopefully, avid for titbits which might be turned into juicy copy. In the Health Service good news is no news. There are three consultants, one GP, and one nurse on the authority, the officers are in attendance at meetings, but the other members' knowledge of health service affairs is limited to what they pick up as they go along. One is a TUC nominee and five are appointed by the City or County Council.

The Chief Executive rules over an empire which is divided into two separate kingdoms, the RI and the rest. Each has its own general manager with its own infrastructure and its own budget, the RI voraciously devouring the lion's share of the District's cash. As the Manager of the Community, Mental Health, Care of the Elderly, and the Children's Unit somewhat ruefully put it, 'You cannot share a bone with a tiger: you either shoot the tiger, or give it the bone'.

It might be thought that all this organizational detail impinges little on the public. To a large extent this is true, although there is a body called the Community Health Council (CHC) in each district which exists to act as a kind of watchdog for the consumer. The secretary is a paid employee, the remainder are local citizens who spend a great deal of time conscientiously scrutinizing the extent to which the Health Authority fulfils its commitments and delivers the goods. Waiting times in clinics, waiting lists, individual complaints, the cleaning standards in the RI are all grist to the mill of the CHC.

The other area in which administration and patients come into fairly direct contact is down at the 'coal face'. The booking clerks in the out-patient clinics are all a part of the medical records personnel, and this is a large and vital component of the machinery which keeps the RI running. The total staff of the department is 300, of whom 100 are medical secretaries. It would be more accurate to state that 100 should be medical secretaries, but at the moment we are seriously understaffed because of the abysmal salaries offered by the hospital service which are currently about £4400 to £5300 with a possible increase to about £6500 for an experienced girl if her post fulfils certain criteria. The duties of the medical secretary extend far beyond typing letters about patients and include dealing tactfully with telephone calls from relatives and GPs, drawing up on-call rotas for junior doctors, arranging major conferences and various meetings, and generally being the focal point of the department and holding it together—to say nothing of pointing the consultants in the right direction at the right time. After a year or so training in my unit, a promising 19-year-old was offered £7250 by a pharmaceutical manufacturer, a salary far higher than her devoted and very experienced superior at the RI.

The other records staff look after the case notes. The numbers on the folders started at one when the NHS was born in 1948 and has now reached about 800 000 and rises by 36 000 each year. The records library can be imagined: it covers the area of a tennis court with a further Olympic-sized swimming pool in the basement for the more ancient folders. A system for putting all case notes and reports on micro-film eight years after last attendance and destroying the file is under active consideration as we are rapidly running out of room. Currently, notes are kept for ever, even when their owner is long dead. The simultaneous introduction of X-ray miniaturization down to 50 mm or so would liberate further space and is also likely to go ahead despite objections from a number of my colleagues.

The movement of case notes around the hospital and keeping track of them and ensuring correct patient identification is a major headache. A degree of relief, comparable to an aspirin, has been obtained from a room full of patient administration system computers, with 32 terminals or VDUs throughout the department. Computers, however, are better at giving orders than actually doing the leg work, and from 6 p.m. until 9 p.m. an army of five filing clerks come in to restore order from the day's chaos. There is also a night-clerk to unearth the vital case record of any patient admitted as an emergency with a previously relevant medical history. The medical records department despatches 500 letters daily to GPs about our patients. It maintains a waiting list of 5500–6000 patients waiting for first appointments, and some 55 000 future appointments which have been registered.

The records officer is also responsible for the bed bureau, who send for patients from the waiting list for admission. They give the patient six weeks' notice but are sometimes unable to honour their promises and so advise the patient to phone in first to make sure the bed is still available. Total daily admissions vary from 20 to 100, the majority of which are emergencies. If the number of available beds through the hospital (excluding maternity and children) falls below 17, a red alert is announced and all 'cold' or elective admissions are cancelled and anyone who can be discharged (the 'Walking Wounded') is despatched home. I recall one occasion when we were down to 10 beds during a hard winter with an outbreak of 'flu when we relied heavily on the goodwill of neighbouring, less sorely pressed, hospitals 20 miles or so distant.

To sound an all too familiar note, two-thirds of the staff of the medical records department are paid below the official government poverty line. A clerk in his or her twenties or early-thirties will probably earn £3700–£4500 a year. You have to rely on your spouse's earnings to live on that, so once again we are short-staffed. The RI continues to function simply because of the amazing loyalty and goodwill of all the people who work in it, and the public and the consultants and the managers would do well to bear the fact constantly in mind.

How far the committee structure has been trimmed by the eagle-eyed scrutiny of the new breed of managers is debatable. At the RI we have a boardroom suite with an additional three committee rooms. The boardroom is in use for meetings for about half the working week together with a number of evenings. The committee rooms are occupied 80 per cent of the time. Not to mention all the others which are held in the medical school, in the seminar rooms, in offices and case conference rooms throughout the complex, day in and day out. They are all very well if that is your line of business, but for the consultants who have to delegate their ward rounds and out-patient clinics they need to be self-evidently important and worthwhile. Very few of them fulfil those criteria. The director of administration estimates that we have at least 40 standing committees or groups who meet regularly on site. By way of example, I personally sit on nine committees, but one is a university function, one is a national committee concerning my specialty, and one is Regional. It is undeniably pleasant to have the opportunity to meet colleagues, but difficult to deny the uncomfortable accuracy of the definition of a committee as 'a cul-de-sac down which good ideas are lured and then quietly strangled'.

14

The lowest form of life:
The medical school

Medical students have come a long way from the good-natured philistines who devoted their time and energy to playing practical jokes, seducing nurses, and damaging their none-too robust brains by a combination of rugger and beer, so vividly portrayed by Richard Gordon in *Doctor in the house* a generation ago. In those far-off days, the principal qualification required in order to secure a place in medical school was a father who could support you through five penurious years and preferably for a few very low-income years thereafter. Nowadays, the places are keenly contested and competition is fiercer than it is for almost any other faculty. Almost, but not quite, because it is easier to pass through the eye of a needle than it is to enter the kingdom of veterinary medicine. To be accepted for training by our sister profession the entry requirement is likely to be three Grade As in the 'A'-levels, in addition to outstanding personal qualities. This is rather curious because most veterinary surgeons qualify and then settle down to practice without much further participation in academic life, whereas all doctors undergo further formal training after qualification, most take higher examinations, and a high proportion undertake research and writing. Perhaps this is in itself a reason for the unattainable standards of veterinary medicine, or perhaps it is something to do with restricting the number of places to the number of veterinary surgeons the animal-owning public will support in the manner to which they have become accustomed. Perhaps it is to do with educational grants for long courses. The hospital doctors, on the other hand, who are mainly salaried, have, until the recent threat of medical unemployment, had few qualms about building new empires and starting new medical schools and expanding old ones. Nevertheless, the demand from sixth formers remains insatiable, and the academic requirements are probably second only to those of the veterinarians.

Is this a good way of choosing future doctors? Surely there are other, more important qualities than intellectual attainment that we should be looking for, such as compassion, commitment, common sense, industry, perhaps even a simple capacity to make people feel better? Perhaps by choosing the academic cream and then offering them a prolonged university education we are merely encouraging them to expect lives of endless intellectual stimulation and opportunities for creativity, when many of the jobs that actually need doing in medicine involve a great deal of routine work which has to be done conscientiously and caringly. I can hear the dean of the medical school at the RI reflecting wearily on these points. His social life consists of dinner parties where he is either attacked on these grounds by the anti-élitist intellectuals of the left, or on the grounds of the insufficiently academic content of clinical medicine by the unashamedly élitist (on the basis that élite means academic which often means of no conceivable practical value) intellectuals of the university. Often he is attacked on both grounds simultaneously, sometimes by the same people. His reply is difficult to dismiss. 'Go for the academic high-fliers', he will say, 'and there are so many of them that you can then select those with the personal qualities you are looking for—if you believe it is possible to detect them at the age of 17. Those you select will then be able to get through their exams as well as playing the clarinet, batting for the cricket eleven, and organizing a voluntary night-sitting service for the sick aged in their own homes throughout the city.' This approach has paid handsome dividends in terms of the articulate, gifted, and committed girls and boys who grace the medical school and give to it as well as taking from it and who go on to a rich variety of careers that reflect credit on the school and the hospital. 'Which of us', the consultants are fond of asking each other (purely rhetorically), 'would stand a chance of getting into medical school today?' I am sure that today's embryo doctors still have a great deal of fun along the way. Although, perhaps there are fewer academics today who are as easy to make fun of as my own aged professor of pathology who lectured in front of a human skeleton which, every time he turned his back, was wired to raise its clanking right upper limb in a solemn salute. However, the parties and the pantomimes go on, and the jokes are still preoccupied with the more fundamental biological activities, despite the superior brain power of their perpetrators.

In terms of practical politics, good 'O'-and 'A'- level grades are the *sine qua non*. The subjects taken at 'A'-level will almost invariably include physics and chemistry, and although most medical schools regard biology as the most desirable third subject, they are almost equally happy if it is mathematics instead. The grades demanded depend on the desirability of the candidate to the medical school, an average offer probably being three B grades. Curiously, it is among the prestigious London teaching hospitals that the most modest demands are made and two of them often make offers of places conditional on gaining three C grades, but they tend to make these offers to applicants who they are fairly confident will, in the event, turn in considerably better grades. Thus, the fact that in 1985, 3907 applicants were accepted from a field of 9839, in the United Kingdom, should not afford too much encouragement to the aspiring medical student as the field was already restricted by self-selection to those whose qualifications gave them a fair chance. Despite a slight decline in popularity compared with law during the past year or two, medicine retains its position among the most highly sought-after university courses.

The offer of a place is made on the basis of reasonable expectations of 'A'-level success, based partly on 'O'-level results and partly on the teachers' assessments, and on the basis of an interview and the information disclosed in the UCCA form. This means that today's youngsters are expected to have *curricula* before they have a chance to have a *vita*. The rules of the game are that it is reasonable to expect candidates to have taken pains to find out something about what they are letting themselves in for and to have founded their choice of career on a realistic view of what the job is all about. Preference will therefore be given to those who have had the initiative to undertake some voluntary work in a hospital or who have taken other steps to enable them to observe some aspect of healthcare at first hand.

As a result of this selection process, the start of each academic year sees 120 new faces at the RI Medical School, of which 50 or 60 are likely to be female. For the first two or three years of the course, they do not really impinge on the life of the institution at all since they are restricted to lecture theatres, dissecting room, and biochemistry and physiology laboratories. After the unrelenting grind of 'A'-levels there is quite an initial thrill in finding yourself dissecting a human body instead of a frog (once the inevitable nausea has been overcome), but it does not last very long: it has to be said that the preclinical years also rapidly become an unrelenting grind and that the light often seems to be flickering rather feebly at the end of an interminable tunnel. The object of dissection is to find out how the body is constructed and to tease out its constituent parts. By this means, assisted by massive texts, copiously illustrated manuals, and numerous lectures and tutorials, a knowledge of anatomy is acquired. Eventually, the precise course and destination of the endless branching network of nerves and blood-vessels are memorized, together with the detailed spatial relationships of muscles, bones, and internal organs— making a simple two-dimensional map of the streets of greater London look the easiest thing in the world to commit to memory by comparison. The microscopic structure of the tissues and their development are included in the course, while the way things work, nerves, muscles, heart, lungs, intestines, liver, and kidneys, form the study of physiology. Biochemistry comprises the complex chemical reactions going on inside the cells to release energy and to transform the dietary nutrients into building blocks and batteries. During the first year the students also learn the way drugs modify the function of the various organs, and they do a course in social medicine. First-year exams are difficult: the second-year exams (second MB) only marginally less so. Once selected, only about 7 per cent of students fail to qualify sooner or later, the majority of the wastage occurring during the preclinical years. The two-year course on normal human biology qualifies the student to proceed to the three-year clinical course. Some 10 per cent elect, instead, to spend a year studying and researching one specialized field of basic science for an honours BSc before doing so. Prolonging the medical course in this way has always proved unattractive to the local education authorities, so financial support has usually come from the Medical Research Council (MRC), a source which at the time of writing, looks in grave danger of drying up.

Two or three years after leaving school, the students are at last set loose on the unsuspecting public. At the RI they wear short white coats to emphasize their traditional status as the lowest form of life. As well as white coats, they wear stethoscopes, at first self-consciously but soon with studied nonchalance. The men are expected to wear ties, look reasonably clean and tidy, and to conduct themselves decorously when on the wards. They are given lectures on ethics and on the standards of behaviour appropriate to apprentice doctors, since most of the teaching is now by apprenticeship. There are still lectures, tutorials and demonstrations, and there is a great deal of reading to do, but most of the time is spent attached to various wards and departments, examining patients, going to theatre, attending post-mortems, and being taken by one of the qualified staff in groups of three or five to be taught on one of the patients. The vast majority of the patients, it should be added, are extraordinarily obliging and readily submit to successive probings and proddings, although they naturally have the right to refuse. The clinical course is rewarding but it also has its frustrations. The student now only has six weeks' holidays a year and spends long days and evenings in the hospital, but he has the compensation of a very pleasant elective period of six weeks in his second year to observe medicine in any location of his choice. We actually receive a number of overseas students who choose to spend their elective period with us, because medical education in the United Kingdom, with its emphasis on contact with patients and on small group bedside teaching is vastly superior to anything on offer, for instance, in Germany. In spite of this, the student is not yet quite a part of the team. He comes on to the ward to examine his patient only to discover that the nurses are doing much more important things to her, or that she is down in the X-ray department, or has visitors. The first time he takes blood it is quite satisfying but then he longs to drain the fluid from a chest or perhaps perform an appendicectomy. A student makes no decision affecting treatment: he may, however, find that he is 'talked through' one or two of these procedures by a friendly registrar. This is particularly likely during attachments to other hospitals in the region. He will almost certainly stitch up a few drunks in A&E after careless mishaps with broken beer bottles. He will compete with the pupil midwives to deliver a few babies. After the day's work he will perhaps seek the sanctuary of the medical school bar, or he will pursue his studies, his musical or sporting interests, or the nurses. Life changes in such a way as to disadvantage one relentlessly. As a student in a London teaching hospital in the 1950s, I and my contemporaries used to be kept hanging about for an hour until the chief turned up, irritable and preoccupied, from Harley Street. He subsequently sent in reports about us to the dean. Now, as a consultant, I turn up on time to my teaching sessions and am kept waiting by the students who then go and report on my performance to the dean (only nowadays it is called 'feedback').

The dean of the medical school is responsible for selecting the students, organizing them through their course, making sure they receive a little exposure to everything of any importance, and achieving a high first-time pass rate at the end. He is a consultant anaesthetist the other half of his working week but had to drop much of his clinical work when the university was pleased to approve his application for the post of dean. He is 'prime minister' of the medical school and is responsible for the £80K per year its library spends on subscriptions to somewhere in excess of 900 different journals for the students and the doctors (Table 14.1). He likes to regard himself as

TABLE 14.1 A specialist's regular reading matter

JOURNALS RECEIVED
British Medical Journal (weekly)
Lancet (weekly)
Hospital Doctor (weekly highly informative 'glossy')
British Journal of Hospital Medicine (monthly)
Prescribers Journal (two-monthly from DHSS)
Drug and Therapeutics Bulletin (bi-monthly from Consumers Association)
Journal of Royal College of Physicians (quarterly)
Hospital Update (monthly)
RI house journal (occasional publication)
Three specialty journals: one quarterly (UK), one quarterly (US), one 'glossy'

JOURNALS REFERRED TO REGULARLY IN THE RI LIBRARY
New England Journal of Medicine (weekly)
Quarterly Journal of Medicine
Postgraduate Medical Journal
Proceedings of the Royal Society of Medicine
A US specialist journal

BOOKS
Progress in . . . . and *Recent advances in* . . . ., which are published every few years. These books are dipped into rather than read cover to cover.

One is also kept up to date by two or three lectures or clinical presentations a week, and by information passed on informally by one's senior registrar.

the social worker to whom a student tormented by dire financial straits or self-doubt or ill-health will turn for counselling, although in practice his flock tend to identify him too closely with the establishment to reveal their weaknesses to him. Instead, they may confide in their supervisors who are doctors in training and therefore still themselves struggling to a greater or lesser degree. It is the dean who answers to the university and to the General Medical Council (GMC) for the quality of the clinical education. The 'king' of the medical school is the professor of medicine and he is responsible for ensuring an adequate performance in terms of research output by the academic (university-employed) doctors, for this weighs heavily with the University Grants Committee (UGC) during their deliberations concerning the financial support they will grant this very expensive part of the university and how many of the nation's quota of medical students we are allowed to admit.

Research is thus almost as integral a part of the RI as teaching, and indeed research is carried out in most hospitals although it is increasingly funded by 'soft money' from a pharmaceutical company or foundation. In every hospital the patients are protected by an Ethical Committee which has lay as well as medical members sitting on it and which scrutinizes each and every project and ensures that all patients undergoing any kind of experiment have given their informed consent. The system works well, given that research has to go on, a premise that few would deny.

This ethical commitment has, at the RI, replaced the old Hippocratic oath. We have no ancient or picturesque traditions. We set papers in medicine, surgery, pathology, obstetrics, and gynaecology, we include questions on psychiatry and pharmacology, we ask the fledgling doctors to examine patients while we observe their technique, we hand them pots containing bits and pieces of pickled disease to identify. When the board of examiners has met and conferred and dined, the time is apt for the university to award them the accolade of Batchelor of Medicine and Batchelor of Surgery and shortly afterwards we take them back as pre-registration house physicians and house surgeons. Which is when they start learning what hard work really means.

15

VIPs or cattle?
The patients

Throughout this book it has been somewhat taken for granted that the entire edifice of the RI together with all its plant, all its equipment and all its staff exists for one purpose only, and that is to serve its patients. Although this statement may smack of the blindingly obvious, it nevertheless needs to be emphatically repeated again and again. The hospital service does not exist to provide glory and research material for the doctors, a trade outlet for the drug industry, or jobs for the domestic staff. It is there to cure sickness when it can, to relieve distress, discomfort, and pain when it cannot cure, to reassure the sick and their families, and to look after the needs of the temporarily incapacitated. There is no shadow of a doubt who are the most important people in any hospital, be it an exorbitantly expensive West End private clinic, a prestigious NHS university hospital, or a dismal, dilapidated, cursorily renovated former workhouse for the long-term elderly sick. The most important people are the patients and they should be made to feel like VIPs even if many of them complain that in practice they are made to feel much more like cattle being herded from one pasture to another, left there to graze for hours on end, and then herded off elsewhere with very little explanation where or why. Pressure, fatigue, and overwork are no excuse for the junior doctor who proceeds to examine a bewildered and apprehensive patient without even having the manners to introduce himself, or for the nurse who resorts to terms of gross familiarity. Innumerable commitments do not entitle a consultant to give less than his entire attention to an undistinguished patient with a pedestrian disease. These are the kinds of thoughtless behaviour that justifiably earn odium for the service as a whole even though such examples are entirely the exception rather than the rule. In general, the hospital service seems to be held in high regard by the British people, the nurses certainly, and perhaps even the doctors to some extent, enjoy a special place in public affection. This affection and confidence makes our role a uniquely privileged one. A personal impression would be that for every patient who lodges a complaint about the way he has been treated in a British hospital, there are half a dozen who feel that it has done its best even though not always very efficiently, and even though they have perhaps been kept waiting around at some inconvenience to themselves. There are probably many more who feel that they have been treated with more courtesy, compassion, and skill than the surroundings had led them to expect.

Who are the patients who throng the out-patient clinics, the halls and the wards of the RI every day, every month, every year? Let it be said first of all that we are witnessing the passing of a breed who will shortly become extinct. There are still stoical old codgers and tough-spirited old birds both from the villages and the city who come in under protest, even though at death's door, never having been in the place before. However, now that all (or almost all) babies are born in hospital, and all (or almost all) mothers are confined in hospital, it is virtually impossible to go through life without having a number on our computer. Everybody is a patient sooner or later, and most people, both sooner and later.

One of the crassly apalling defects in the system which applies to virtually all hospitals is that as far as the DHSS is concerned, it does not appear to matter whether a patient dies or goes home from hospital. The figures are all lumped together under the heading 'deaths and discharges' and it is extraordinarily difficult to separate the two. In the year ending 31 December 1985 the total number of deaths and discharges from the RI was, in round figures, 29 500. This represents a 9% per cent increase over the total for 1980, and a breakdown for the main specialties is given in Table 15.1 Specialties vary enormously in the relative use they make of out-patient or day-case treatment compared with in-patient care, and also, among the admissions, how many are emergencies and how many are planned admissions. The pattern of routine admissions also varies widely, and some specialties such as ENT habitually bring people in the day before the regular operating list and discharge them a day or so afterwards except for a relatively small number of major cases. The average duration of stay for a scatter of different specialties is therefore given in Table 15.2 These tables give some idea of the utilization of the hospital beds by different categories of patient.

Table 15.3 gives a surprisingly different picture, the main reasons why all these patients came to be admitted in the first place. The leading one, concussion, is a loose diagnosis covering a multitude of different degrees of severity of head injury, many of them including

TABLE 15.1 Deaths and discharges by main
specialty, excluding maternity, (year ending
31 December 1985, figures rounded)

Medical specialties*	7600
Neurology	700
Paediatrics	1500
Dental surgery	500
ENT	1700
Ophthalmology	1700
General surgery	4000
Gynaecology	2600
Neurosurgery	1800
Orthopaedics and trauma	2400
Urology	2100
Plastic surgery	900
Transplant surgery	250
Radiotherapy	1600
Other	150
Total	*29 500*

* General medicine, geriatric medicine, haematology,
cardiology, respiratory medicine, dermatology, infectious
diseases, rheumatology and rehabilitation, nephrology.

TABLE 15.2 Average duration of stay (days)
for various specialties (year ending 31
December 1985)

General medicine	10.7
Geriatric medicine (acute)	18.7
Paediatrics	4.7
Rheumatology and rehabilitation	22.0
Dermatology	21.0
Dental surgery	2.6
ENT	3.6
General surgery	6.3
Gynaecology	4.1
Neurosurgery	9.5
Ophthalmology	4.6
Orthopaedics and trauma	11.6
Radiotherapy	10.9
Urology	4.9
Overall average stay per patient	*8.5*

little more than overnight observation to pick up the very occasional
catastrophic intracranial bleeding requiring surgical evacuation to
decompress the brain. Table 15.4 gives yet another side of the story: if
you walk up to a bed, what is the occupant likely to have wrong with

TABLE 15.3 Main causes of admission (1984)

Diagnosis	No.	% of all admissions
Concussion	949	3.3
Legal termination of pregnancy	659	2.3
Sterilization	614	2.1
Disorders of menstruation	592	2.1
Cerebrovascular disease	588	2.1
Abdominal hernias	567	2.0
Non-specific symptoms of abdomen and pelvis	552	1.9
Coronary heart disease	528	1.8
Diseases of the pulmonary circulation and other forms of heart disease	492	1.7
Cancer of the bladder	461	1.6
Cataract	457	1.6
Disorders of tooth development and eruption	387	1.4
Retinal detachment and defects	349	1.2
Symptoms involving the urinary system	333	1.2
Chronic disease of tonsils and adenoids	312	1.1
Appendicitis	307	1.1
Fractured neck of femur	301	1.1
General symptoms (includes coma, convulsions)	292	1.0
Gallstones and other diseases of the biliary tract	291	1.0
Other diseases of urethra and urinary tract	291	1.0
All other causes	19 274	67.4

Source: Hospital Activity Analysis.

him or her? A complicated pattern is beginning to emerge which suggests, not very surprisingly, that there are going to be considerable differences in the type of person admitted briefly after a rugger injury and one who occupies a bed for many weeks due to a stroke. One obvious difference is in age, and some data on this subject are presented in Table 15.5. Table 15.6 indicates the bed-mix of the RI as it is nominally constituted at present.

It is apparent that in the late-twentieth century, in Western countries, there is a very high tendency for sickness to be something that afflicts the elderly. Broadly speaking, the over 65-year-olds who comprise only 15 per cent of the population utilize over half of the general medical beds, almost half of the general surgical beds, about half of the orthopaedic beds, and about 45 per cent of all acute beds. (They also, incidentally occupy about half of the psychiatric beds.) Fractures in the region of the hip, for instance, are a major epidemic of our times and are increasing in prevalence out of proportion to the general ageing of society. By the age of 85, almost 15 per cent of women will have sustained a fracture of the neck of the femur and

TABLE 15.4 Main causes of bed utilization (1984 excluding maternity)

Diagnosis	Daily occupied beds	% of all occupied beds
Cerebrovascular disease	40	6.5
Fractured neck of femur	22	3.4
Diseases of the pulmonary circulation and other forms of heart disease	16.5	2.7
Concussion	15	2.4
Coronary heart disease	15	2.4
Diabetes mellitus	10	1.6
Colorectal cancer	9	1.5
Cancer of the breast	8.5	1.4
Malignant neoplasm of brain	8	1.4
Gallstones and other biliary tract diseases	8	1.3
Hernia of the abdominal cavity	7.5	1.2
Chronic renal failure	7.5	1.2
Pneumonia and influenza	7	1.2
Cancer of the bladder	6.5	1.1
Cataract	6.5	1.1
Fracture of other parts of femur	6.5	1.1
Non-psychotic mental disorders with special symptoms not elsewhere classified	6.5	1.1
Osteoarthrosis and allied disorders	6	1.0
Intervertebral disc disorders	6	1.0
Hyperplasia of prostate	6	1.0
All other causes	396	64.4

Source: Hospital Activity Analysis.

TABLE 15.5 Average percentage of beds occupied daily by age group in various specialties (England, 1983)

	Total bed number	% of occupants in age range					
		0–4	5–14	15–44	45–64	65–74	75–84	85+
General medicine	23 613			11.3	31	28	22.3	6.5
General surgery	19 638	1.7	3.2	18.7	28.3	23.9	19.7	4.4
Traumatic and orthopaedic surgery	15 901	2.1	6	25	18.5	16	21.5	10.8
Gynaecology	6479			60.8	24.8	8.2	4.3	1.3
Geriatric medicine	49 723				4	18.8	46.8	30.5
All specialties other than psychiatry	151 437	3.75	2.9	13	18.7	19.9	27.4	14
General population	46.846 million	6.3	13	43	22.3	8.9	5	1

Source: Hospital In-Patient Enquiry

TABLE 15.6 Nominal designation of beds by specialty (round figures)

General medicine	110
Paediatrics	25
Dermatology	15
Neurology	20
Rheumatology and rehabilitation	30
Geriatrics	65
Haematology	15
Infectious diseases	10
Nephrology	10
General surgery	90
Paediatric surgery including eye, ENT, Urology, plastic etc.	35
Transplant surgery	5
Cardiothoracic medicine and surgery	30
ENT	25
Trauma and orthopaedics	90
Ophthalmology	30
Urology	35
Plastic surgery including burns	20
Dental surgery	10
Neurosurgery	50
Gynaecology	40
Obstetrics	95
Special care baby unit	20
ITU, CCU	15
Radiotherapy	60
Total	*950*

more women die as a result of this injury and its complications than of cancer of the breast, womb, and neck of the womb combined. Old men make considerable demands on surgical services also, of course: it has been estimated that a 40-year-old man has a 10 per cent chance of requiring a prostatectomy by the time he reaches the age of 80. In addition, the old have exclusive access to all those geriatric beds. The ills that ageing flesh is heir to are the major challenge facing medicine in the developed nations as the century draws to its close. Sometimes they can be cured, usually they can be relieved, and an equally important aim is the preservation of activity and independence in old age by active rehabilitation as soon as the acute phase of the illness has been treated. 'We are all geriatricians now' is a commonly heard saying in the corridors of our hospitals, and anyone who does not enjoy dealing with the old and their problems would be well advised to think twice before taking up medicine or nursing as a profession.

Having addressed the questions of why the patients are in hospital and who they are, perhaps we should attempt to find out what happens to them once they are in. To start on a fairly minor note, albeit an uncomfortable one, it appears that 10 or 12 per cent of all patients admitted have a catheter passed into the bladder at some time during their stay. More seriously, pressure sores affect some 5 per cent of all patients in a DGH, but although the hospital is often blamed for this occurrence, it has to be said that the seeds are often sown before admission and a frail and aged subject who has been lying helpless on the floor at home following a fall is very likely to have sustained tissue damage even if there is not an open sore by the time he or she is admitted. Nowadays, people are kept in bed for the absolute minimum period of time, only as long, in fact, as they feel too awful to get up, and bed rest is scarcely ever prescribed as a treatment. It was a form of treatment greatly beloved by the physicians of a generation ago, until Richard Asher, an eminent London physician of the 1950s and 1960s, drew the attention of the medical world to the grave dangers of lying in bed. Nowadays, the emphasis is on mobilization, and do not imagine that you go into hospital for a rest.

In any case, nothing is less conducive to a rest than the bustle of a hospital ward, and this was graphically illustrated by a young American physician who had the misfortune to be admitted to her own hospital with a not particularly grave complaint. She kept a diary of the number of members of staff she came into contact with during the course of their duties, and there is no reason to suppose that the experience in a British hospital would be significantly different from that recorded in her transatlantic chronicle. The number of these contacts was greatest on Monday (69) and least on Sunday (34). On the Monday, 37 of them were with nursing staff, 20 with medical staff, seven were with auxiliaries, four with housekeeping personnel, one miscellaneous: she received, in addition, six visitors that day. The contacts with staff occurred when they entered her room or when she was taken to a diagnostic facility. During a five-day stay, she was only able to take one two-hour nap between 7 a.m. and 10 p.m. and she concluded that if it is a rest you are after, you would do far better to stay in an hotel.

To turn to the more major events that befall people admitted to hospital, something like a third of the elderly patients on a general surgical ward come in as emergencies and about a half undergo operations. Which brings us to the popularity rating of the different kinds of surgical operation available, both emergency and elective: the current top 10 are given in Table 15.7. Total NHS operations are given and an estimated number which would occur in a DGH serving a population of 250 000.

TABLE 15.7 Number of different categories of surgical operations performed in NHS hospitals (England, 1984)

Operation	Total NHS	DGH
D&C, biopsy, and excision of lesions of cervix	116 780	620
Surgical treatment of fractures	95 300	510
Cystoscopy and treatment of bladder lesion	86 330	455
Tonsils and adenoids	77 620	415
Hysterectomy	65 860	350
Inguinal hernia repair	64 400	340
Abdominal surgery	64 370	340
Post-natal, post-abortion	60 540	320
Operations on teeth, gums, and jaws (excluding abscesses and simple extractions)	59 800	315
Operations on lens of eye (e.g. cataract)	55 270	290
All others	1 505 550	8000
Total	2 251 820	11 900

Source: Hospital In-patient Enquiry.

Perhaps the biggest anxiety either consciously or subconsciously harboured by anyone going into hospital is the simple fear 'am I going to die?' The chances of such an outcome can perhaps be gauged by the fact that the 29 500 deaths and discharges from the RI during 1985 included 1130 deaths which was about 3.4 per cent of the total. Even in the geriatric wards, the proportion of deaths is only 17.5 per cent of the admissions. Here, it must be remembered, considerable numbers of patients are sent in simply because the GP thinks they probably have an inevitably fatal illness and would look after them at home if it were possible to keep them comfortable and well cared for. Increasingly, deaths do take place in hospital and the public has come to regard hospital as the proper place for all anticipated deaths, which is somewhat illogical since most of us would much prefer to die in our own homes. Nevertheless, 62:5 per cent of all deaths in England and Wales in 1984 took place in hospitals, the remainder occurring in private households, public places, and old peoples' homes. The figures quoted, however, should offer some reassurance that death is a most unlikely outcome of your hospital admission.

Finally, are the public appreciative of their hospital and the care it gives them? My ward sister reckons that 70 per cent of her patients, or their families, produce material evidence of their gratitude on their departure in the form of a card or a letter, or some flowers or chocolates for the nurses. Even more impressively, the trust funds receive donations of £300K a year and legacies of £140K, and many more gifts are made to individual research funds. The other side of the coin is the number of complaints lodged with the Health Authority. These would overwhelmingly concern the real or imagined short-comings of the RI although a small minority would relate to grievances against the other hospitals in the District. In 1983 there were 135 such complaints, in 1984 there were 140, and in 1985, 165. The majority are fairly easily dealt with by the management, or by the senior nurses, or by a letter of reassurance from the consultant. Occasionally, in 20 or 30 cases a year, legal advice has to be sought, and a very, very few—one or two a year—go to an independent committee of enquiry or to the Health Service Commissioner (the Ombudsman). The less serious complaints are often concerned with the delays that seem to be an inescapable part of the hospital scene. For example, the CHC conducted a survey of the clinics and found that 44 per cent of patients were kept waiting over 30 minutes and 16 per cent, over an hour: six clinics had over 25 per cent of their patients delayed an hour or more.

Being kept waiting may be an inconvenience, but far more serious are the effects of delays due to long waiting lists. From time to time, politicians issue statements about the numbers of people in the United Kingdom on hospital waiting-lists. These numbers make little impact, because they have the indigestibility of the proverbial telephone numbers, and because who cares anyway? What matters is not how many people there are on the waiting list, but how long they have to wait while the disease becomes more serious or they suffer unnecessary pain. Waiting lists build up in those specialties where they are tolerable. You cannot have a waiting list for a confinement, a fracture, or for the admission of the acutely sick. It is in the field of elective surgery that there are traditionally delays before seeing the specialist in clinic, and then before being sent for to come in. At the RI the waiting time for a routine eye appointment is four months for one ophthalmologist, 10 months for another. The situation in ENT and orthopaedic surgery is similar. For patients accepted for cataract extraction or total hip replacement, there is the second period of waiting which may be a year or two, and for the socially if not medically desirable procedure of vasectomy, you may have to wait 15 months. The actual waiting list for orthopaedic surgery is currently about 1650 out of a total in-patient waiting list of 5300. It is simply very difficult to squeeze-in 'routine' surgery when the place is invariably awash with trauma. Small wonder that irritation may cloud the eventual consultation, and perhaps it is a matter of surprise that the complaints although increasing in numbers, are only keeping pace with the throughput of patients.

This is the final point which needs to be made about our patients: they keep on coming. Almost whatever aspect of the work of the RI you examine, it seems to be increasing at a rate of about 5 per cent a year. Medical admissions, X-rays, cancer clinics, fractures; the story is the same for almost every department and every specialty. However, our catchment population is not growing. The city and our other towns and villages have been in a stable state of zero population growth for the past 25 years. So, why, when we are working so hard to make people better, are they obstinately becoming progressively sicker? When the NHS was first established, the politicians of the day seriously thought that the workload would soar in its early years as people learned how to use it and the unreported disease in the community surfaced, but would then decline once the existing burden of illness had declared itself and had been dealt with. In 1987 that view looks extremely naive, and no politician knows how to fuel the continuously accelerating engines of the hospital service. The reasons why hospital medicine remains a growth industry are not entirely clear, but there are probably several factors at work. One is the ageing of the population: another is the development of new medical techniques: and a third may well be the rising health expectations of the public. While blaming the public, it also has to be said that unhealthy habits persist—tobacco, alcohol, dietary indiscretion, driving around in fast cars and on fast motor bikes, and pursuing hazardous leisure activities. However, it is principally the ageing population that keeps sickness alive and well and likely to remain so for the rest of the century as the numbers of the very old continue to swell, for it is increasingly the case that the NHS lavishes the major part of each individuals's share of its resources on the last six months of his life.

What of the future? It presents the enormous conceptual challenge of bridging the gap between the moderately hard science of statistically sound clinical trials and the structureless anarchy of trying to rationalize the provision of support to the disabled and dependent. The hospital service dispenses attempted cure and immediate care. A great deal of the former is shifting its emphasis from the wards to the community. We have seen the impact of day-case surgery on routine surgical procedures. All elective investigational medicine is now performed on an out-patient basis, the initial clinic attendance being followed by a series of tests which are sometimes carried out in a 'Programmed Investigative Unit' to spare the patient the inconvenience of being boarded in the admittedly rather indifferent hotel facilities on offer at the local hospital. Meanwhile, the wards are flooded with the unceasing tide of emergencies, most of which are sent in for the purpose of basic support. This support may be of a high tech variety, as is the case with major emergency surgery, myocardial infarction, and diabetic coma. Much of it is comparatively unsophisticated. The main reason that so many stroke victims come in as emergencies, however, is not in order to receive CT scan confirmation of the diagnosis or heroically interventional treatment, but simply because there are not enough people at home to administer to their everyday bodily needs. One of the greatest resources at the command of the local DGH is the staff, especially perhaps the nursing staff. The DGH of the future, will do as much of its work as it can in day surgery units and programmed investigational units: its emergency caseload will be divided into low dependency (A&E), high dependency (general medicine, geriatrics), and very high dependency (ITU, CCU, 'high dependency units').

16

Financial 'black hole' or value for money?

How much does it cost to run the hospital and does it give good value for money? The first question can only be answered with surprising difficulty, and the second is heavily dependent on a number of value judgements. The figures are only meaningful if set in the national and international contexts of public expenditure. The annual cost of the health service is certainly growing in terms of pounds sterling (Table 16.1). In real terms, adjusted for inflation, the rise has been almost four-fold since its inception, from £437 million in 1949 to about £1500 million at 1949 prices in 1983. These figures are less impressive when set beside those of comparable nations. The per capita expenditure on health in the United Kingdom is currently £290 per annum, while countries such as Sweden, the United States, Switzerland, France, The Netherlands, and West Germany spend around £400. In a typical year, the way that the NHS budget is divided up is depicted in Fig. 1, which illustrates that the hospital service receives the lion's share of the cake. Figure 2 gives an idea of how the finance is deployed within the hospital service.

The DHSS decides how the NHS budget will be apportioned to the regions, and the RHAs decide how their allocation will be split up among the eight or so districts which they each administer. Our own District currently (1986–7) receives a budget of £65 million because of its special nature: a very small neighbouring District (population 115 000), with a DGH and one or two regional specialties receives £19 million. Few of us believe that the data base is sufficiently sophisticated to permit this distribution to be other than somewhat arbitrary. In fairness to the present government, it has to be said that we received £59 million during 1984–5 and £57 million in 1983–4. Of our £65 million, the amount spent on running the RI is a curiously inaccessible figure, for a variety of reasons. For example, the maternity wing is financially treated as a separate hospital and the nursing budget covers both the community and the psychiatric hospital, hence the proportion spent on the RI is not easy to tease out.

TABLE 16.1 Annual expenditure on the
NHS in the United Kingdom

Year	Cost of NHS (£ million)	% of public expenditure
1978–79	9137	13.9
1985–86	17 429	15
1988–89	24 089 (estimated)	16.2

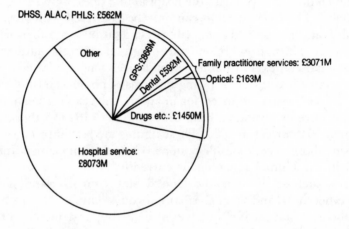

FIG. 1   NHS expenditure, England 1983–84 (total expenditure: £13 147 million).

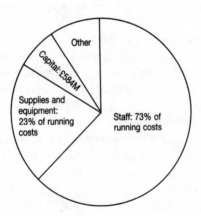

FIG. 2   Hospital service expenditure, England, 1983–84 (total expenditure: £8073 million).

As far as an analysis of the March 1985 figures revealed, the RI accounted for something over £35.5 million during the preceding year, making the running cost over £4K per hour. A further scrutiny of the financial statements yields a variety of information and in the following tables I have placed the RI by comparison with the other five acute hospitals of over 100 beds in the Region. None of the others are teaching hospitals and the regional specialties are heavily, although not exclusively, concentrated on the RI site. The information in Table 16.2 is liable to stir up all sorts of emotion, particularly when some unfortunate patient has completed his treatment but has nowhere to be discharged to and has therefore become a 'bed-blocker' at £100 a day. The fact is that he is actually costing the taxpayer less than £100 but it is the other patients, still on the receiving end of all that high technology, who are costing more, and that if it were not for a few 'bed-blockers' acute hospitals would cost even more than they do. Hospitals like the RI work reasonably efficiently, and in truth there is no available finance for them to increase their activity any further. It is readily admitted that we can only really manage within our budget if some outside event such as a major strike puts a brake on the constant throughput, turnover, operating activity, admission, and discharge through a totally open and staffed hospital.

TABLE 16.2 Costs per patient (1984–85)

	RI (£)	Position in Regional league	Regional average (£)
Cost per in-patient day	100	2	89
(psychiatric hospital:	45		
long-stay geriatric hospital)	33		
Cost per in-patient case	835	1	573
Cost per out-patient attendance*	26	2	23
Cost per A&E attendance	23	1	15

* New cases are far more expensive than follow ups.

Table 16.3 can be viewed in the context that the occupancy for the year was 80 per cent, which was top equal among the six roughly comparable hospitals, and Table 16.4 in the context that the number of new out-patient referrals was 53 600 which put us easily top of the Regional league. There were almost 235 000 out-patient attendances altogether, not counting the ANC, which was again comfortably top of the list. A rough idea of the patient categories using up the

TABLE 16.3 Breakdown of costs per in-patient per day (1984–5)

Service	£	Regional position
Medical staff	10.75	1 (just)
Nursing staff	28.20	4
Medical/surgical supplies	7.00	1 (just)
Pharmacy	7.80	1 (easily)
Other treatment	2.00	5
Radiology	1.80	1
Pathology	3.80	1
Physiotherapy	0.90	2
Administration	7.70	2
Medical records	1.70	2
Catering	3.40	3
Portering	2.45	1
Linen, laundry	1.55	
Engineering	3.50	2
Energy, etc.	4.05	
Building maintenance	1.40	
Estate	2.75	
Other	9.75	
Total	*100.50*	

TABLE 16.4 Breakdown of costs per out-patient attendance (1984–85)

Service	£	Regional position
Medical staff	6.10	1 (just)
Nursing	2.30	3
Supplies	1.50	2
Pharmacy	1.40	1
Radiography	1.55	2
Pathology	1.80	2
Administration	2.00	
Other	9.35	
Total	*26.00*	

resources is given in Table 16.5, and some of the non-professional services are costed in Table 16.6. In addition to the hospital costs, there are certain activities which involve the hospital but are separately funded. The whole Regional Ambulance Service, in 1984–85 for example, cost just over £10.25 million, or £5.30 for every member of the population.

Armed with this bewildering array of figures, it is impossible to answer the question posed by the title of the chapter. Yes, the hospital

TABLE 16.5 Where the money goes, (1984–85, figures rounded)

Type of patient	£ (million)
In-patients	23.5
Out-patients	6.0
A&E	1.0
Day-cases	0.6
Maternity	3.0
Other	1.5
Total	35.6

TABLE 16.6 Annual cost of services (1984–85, figures rounded)

Services	£K
Catering	810*
Boilers	207
Buildings	453
Engineering	1145
Gas, oil, electricity	1021
Radiography	1038
Operating theatres	1825
Intensive care	345
Domestic	1011
Laundry	174
Total	8029

* Includes £1.53 per patient per day on provisions.

costs a great deal, and arguably no, there is not a great deal of wastage and some of the costs have been pared to the bone. It is even difficult to interpret the sums in such a way as to make comparisons. The other Districts in the Region point to high unit costs in the RI. However, the RI does a great deal of Regional and even national work. Because of the reputations of the consultants, patients are sent to them from all over the Region and from neighbouring Regions, not just to the designated regional specialties but into the ordinary DGH specialties, and these patients are likely to be more complicated than the average and to cost more. Meanwhile, the waiting lists grow from our own city inhabitants who need hips replaced and cataracts removed. Both types of work have to be done in a place like the RI with the expertise to do them. Both types of clientele are essential to a great teaching hospital and we do not have the resources to match both tasks. It does not appear particularly likely that much more money will be pumped into the NHS whichever government is in power. It does seem likely that the private sector will continue to thrive. Even there, comparisons are invidious. A private hospital specializing in elective surgery on a small or medium scale should be able to keep its costs down. It does not have any very expensive, major operations, moribund poor-risk salvage procedures, ITU, and training commitment. The staff of the RI may, perhaps, be forgiven for thinking that they are penalized in some respects for being the flagship of the fleet.

These arguments are acquiring a special urgency during 1987 because it is emerging that the Health Authority has accumulated a £2½ million overspend, which means that it needs to claw a substantial proportion of that amount back this year, plus reducing last year's expenditure by almost £1 million this year in order not to do the same again, plus financing inflation (including a hopefully substantial salary increase for the nurses this time round). How can we save almost £3 million? The simple answers are (a) that we cannot do so, (b) that we have to unless we can persuade the Region that we have long been seriously underfunded. We can engender revenue, but most of it is on a fairly minor scale and more grandiose schemes such as the development of a private hospital on the site are fraught with difficulties and disadvantages. We can turn capital into revenue by disposing of some accommodation for nurses scattered around the city, but this is the proverbial 'selling off the family silver' and would have dire consequences next time we were in a position to try to recruit more nurses to a city where property is expensive both to buy and to rent. We can, and will probably have to, postpone starting on such long overdue developments as upgrading or replacing some of the facilities for housing the aged and mentally infirm which are an 'absolute disgrace' (for once, the local newspaper got it right). We will eventually probably have to make cuts—like closing wards and laying-off all our agency nurses. You cannot close the medical or geriatric wards which are full and overflowing into the surgical wards. You have to choose wards where the bulk of the admissions are elective rather than urgent, and where the waiting list is not too long. The medical staff have all been here before and realize there is no light at the end of the tunnel, only another train coming in the opposite direction. Should they be a party to giving advice on these matters? They have to, otherwise a tragic decision will be also a totally irrational one. The position of the hospital manager is even worse. From his point of view, as the American health economist Victor Fuchs wrote as long ago as 1974, 'running a hospital is like trying to drive a car when the passengers have control of the wheel and the accelerator. The most the administrator can do is occasionally jam on the brakes'.

One possibility is to argue with the Region that too much of the local cake goes to the smaller districts with new, expanding hospitals: we, at the centre, are being starved. The argument is similar to the cries of anguish emerging from the London teaching hospitals, those historic institutions which have done so much to make British medicine pre-eminent. During the 1970s the population flowed away from London and the cash became scarcer. The notorious Resource Allocation Working Party (RAWP—as in 'we've been RAWPed') decreed that funds would be diverted from the (comparatively) luxuriously provided capital to the (by any standards) penurious Midlands and North. Now the great and famous hospitals are facing closures of wards, services, medical schools, whole hospitals, and they are, quite rightly, refusing to die without a struggle. At the RI we share their despair. While London is bleating, the RI is bleeding. Eventually, it all comes back to the amount of money we are prepared to spend on health care (Table 16.7).

TABLE 16.7 Annual expenditure per capita on health care (1982)

Country	US dollars
United States	1388
Sweden	1168
France	931
The Netherlands	836
Japan	602
United Kingdom	508
Spain	302
Greece	187

Source: Organization for Economic Cooperation and Development (OECD).

It has to be admitted that the policies of the Conservative government have heightened awareness of the need to improve economic analysis of human activities which cost a great deal but do not readily lend themselves to it, of which healthcare is a prime example. We have more able minds focusing on healthcare delivery than ever before. What they have come up with is the Quality Adjusted Life Year, or QALY. One positive QALY is a year of life free from pain, distress, and disability. A year of life lived in such severe pain or dependency that the subject would rather be dead (which is rated zero) could be a negative QALY. No one can say how much a QALY is worth, but they are busy working out how much it costs and allocating higher priority to activities with a low cost per QALY. An activity which generates only two QALYs but costs only £200 costs £100 per QALY, but one which generates five QALYs but costs £2000 costs £400 per QALY. A treatment which gives a patient four years of healthy life expectancy in lieu of four years pain or disability rated at 0.75 would result in a gain of $4 \times 0.25 = 1$ QALY, but another treatment which improved the patient from a level of 0.25 to 0.75 for four years would be worth two QALYs. This attempt at quantification remains something of a gleam in its inventor's eye but a few examples of activities relatively easy to work out are given in Table 16.8.

TABLE 16.8 Cost per Quality Adjusted Life Year (QALY)

	£K
Haemo dialysis	9.00
CAPD	13.50
Heart transplant	8.00
Renal transplant	3.50
CABG	2.0
Pacemaker	1.0
THR	0.75
GP's counselling to stop smoking	0.20

There is at present a great deal of pressure from the high command of the NHS to introduce 'clinical management budgeting'. This would allocate to each consultant or head of department his own budget, thereby giving responsibility to those best qualified to exercise it, or shifting the blame for the meagre rationing of inadequate resources depending on one's viewpoint. So far, the pilot trials do not look convincing. One problem is that a clinician such as myself has very little control over his spending. A ward of 28 beds has to have a given number of nurses and doctors, and their salaries are nationally fixed. I have no control over the nature of the medical emergencies admitted, and therefore hardly any over their treatment. A degree of discretion can be exercised over the investigations which my staff request in my name, but they can only amount to about 5 per cent of the cost of the ward. The thought of the extra work involved is an added disincentive, and it is in any case very doubtful if the patients would appreciate the presence of the accountant on the consultant's ward round.

Healthcare, as we have seen, is expensive and sickness care, even more so. The RI is not really in the business of health promotion, but of picking up the pieces when prevention has not worked. The government and the profession emphasize the importance of health education and of preventive medicine. These, together with improved housing, sanitation, nutrition, and general standard of living have achieved more benefits to the overall health of the population of our city than the RI ever did. However, no one ever thanked any official for preventing them from contracting an illness, and it is not even very easy to obtain much job satisfaction from doing so. Everyone expects treatment when sickness or calamity strikes, and no civilized society would tolerate withdrawal of the facilities for providing it. The various departments we have visited exist because we will always have ill health and suffering and because looking after the sick is the world's most satisfying and challenging occupation. To heal some-times, to relieve often, to comfort always, remains the aim of those who work in any hospital.

The activities which we have observed within the walls of the RI are to be found in many similar hospitals which combine the functions of a fairly large DGH and a specialized Regional centre. The figures will vary in accordance with bed numbers and mix between specialties but can be extrapolated to fit other localities and other hospitals with slight variations to take into account differences in scale, social circumstances, and age structure. To those who work there, the RI is special, and many of its patients feel the same way about it. This book has painted as accurate a picture of its inner workings as is possible, given that the subject is an ever moving one. Some of the information will already be out of date by the time it reaches print, but the broad sweep of the canvas and the trends which it portrays will still be valid despite intervening developments and elections. We hope the RI will flourish and expand to enable us to do what we would dearly like to do for our patients. Our sources of information do not encourage optimism on this score given the likely economic climate irrespective of which political party holds power during the remainder of the century.

APPENDIX

Contents of the orange emergency box*

Ventilating bag and mask
Laryngoscope
Endotracheal tubes
Suction catheters
Gauze swabs
Airways
Selection of syringes and needles
200 ml of sodium bicarbonate 8.4%
Foam pack containing the following ampoules:
   Adrenaline 1 mg in 10 ml
   Atropine 0.5 mg in 5 ml
   Aminophylline 250 mg in 10 ml x 2
   Calcium gluconate 10% 10 ml x 2
   Chlorpheniramine 10 mg
   Dextrose 50% 50 ml
   Diazepam emulsion 10 mg x 2
   Frusemide 50 mg in 5 ml x 2
   Hydrocortisone 100 mg x 2
   Lignocaine 1% 10 ml
   Naloxone 400 mcg

* There are probably some 50 of these boxes which are located in all wards and departments throughout the hospital in preparation for a wide range of medical emergencies.

INDEX